70
Herbal Recipes

Natural Methods of Healing

130 images

"70 Herbal Recipes: Natural Methods of Healing" invites you into the enchanting world of herbal medicine and natural wellness. This comprehensive guide offers a collection of **70 powerful recipes** designed to enhance your health, boost your immunity, and support your well-being—all through the gentle yet potent power of herbs.

With **130 vibrant, full-color illustrations**, this book not only provides practical knowledge but also brings the beauty of nature's remedies to life. Each recipe is accompanied by a stunning visual representation, making it easy to identify herbs and follow the preparation process.

What You'll Discover:

- **Simple Recipes**: Step-by-step instructions for creating teas, tinctures, salves, and more.
- **Holistic Guidance**: Insights into using herbs for immunity, digestion, relaxation, energy, and more.
- **Growing and Harvesting Tips**: Advice on cultivating your own herbal garden.
- **Safety First**: Recommendations for safe and effective use of herbal remedies for all ages.

Whether you're an experienced herbalist or a beginner, this book will inspire you to explore the ancient wisdom of plant-based healing and incorporate it into your modern lifestyle.

"70 Herbal Recipes" is more than a recipe book—it's a visual journey into the timeless art of herbal medicine. Let the stunning illustrations and easy-to-follow instructions guide you to natural health and harmony.

Table of Content

Introduction

Welcome to **"70 Herbal Recipes: Natural Methods of Healing,"** a book inspired by the time-honored traditions of herbal medicine and the remarkable healing power of nature. For centuries, people across the world have turned to plants for their therapeutic properties, using them to soothe ailments, strengthen the body, and bring balance to the mind and spirit. This book is your guide to exploring the abundant gifts of the natural world and learning how to integrate herbal remedies into your daily life.

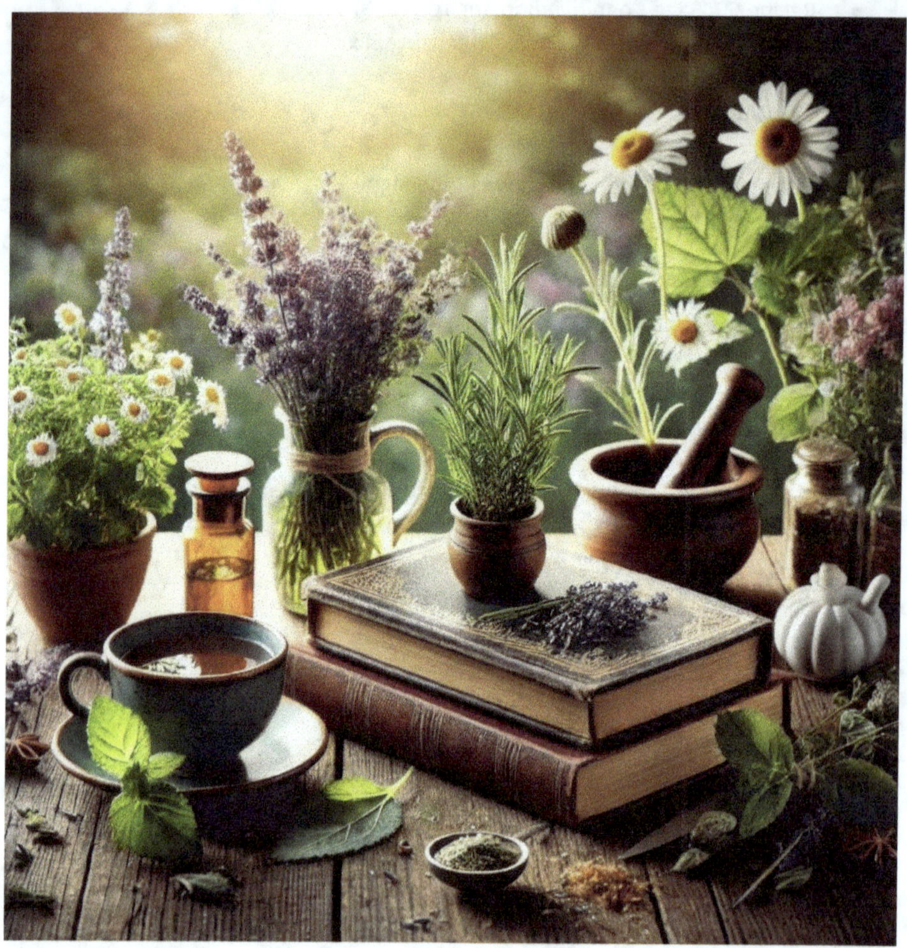

Why Herbs?

In our fast-paced, modern world, it's easy to feel disconnected from nature and overwhelmed by synthetic solutions to common health concerns. Herbs offer an alternative—a gentle, holistic approach that works in harmony with your body. From calming chamomile to invigorating ginger, each plant holds unique properties that can help you achieve greater vitality and well-being.

Herbal medicine is not just about treating symptoms; it's about supporting the body's natural ability to heal itself. Whether you're looking to boost your immune system, ease stress, or care for your skin, herbs provide a wealth of possibilities. With a little knowledge and guidance, you can create your own remedies tailored to your specific needs.

What You'll Find in This Book

This book is a collection of **70 recipes**, each thoughtfully crafted to address different aspects of health and wellness. You'll discover teas, tinctures, salves, syrups, and more—all made from natural, easy-to-find ingredients. Every recipe is accompanied by **a full-color illustration**, ensuring that you can follow the instructions with confidence and clarity.

Here's a glimpse of what you'll learn:

- How to support your immune system with elderberry syrup or echinacea tea.
- Ways to calm your mind and improve sleep with lavender baths and valerian tinctures.
- Gentle remedies for children, like lemon balm popsicles and chamomile syrups.
- Tips for growing, harvesting, and storing your own herbs to ensure a fresh, organic supply.

Who Is This Book For?

This book is for everyone—whether you're an experienced herbalist or just beginning to explore natural remedies. It's for the parents who want gentle solutions for their children, the busy professionals seeking stress relief, and anyone looking to embrace a healthier, more holistic lifestyle.

No special equipment or prior knowledge is required. All you need is a curiosity about the natural world and a desire to reconnect with the wisdom of our ancestors.

A Word of Caution

While herbal remedies can be incredibly powerful, they are not a substitute for professional medical advice. Always consult with a qualified healthcare provider before starting any new herbal regimen, especially if you are pregnant, nursing, or have underlying health conditions.

A Journey Back to Nature

Herbal medicine invites us to slow down, to observe, and to engage with the rhythms of the earth. As you read this book and experiment with its recipes, you'll discover not only the therapeutic power of plants but also a deeper connection to nature and yourself.

So take a moment, breathe deeply, and let this book guide you on a journey of healing and renewal. Whether you're sipping a warm cup of herbal tea or crafting a soothing salve, know that you are partaking in an ancient tradition— one rooted in the wisdom of nature and the resilience of the human spirit.

Welcome to the world of herbal healing. Let's get started.

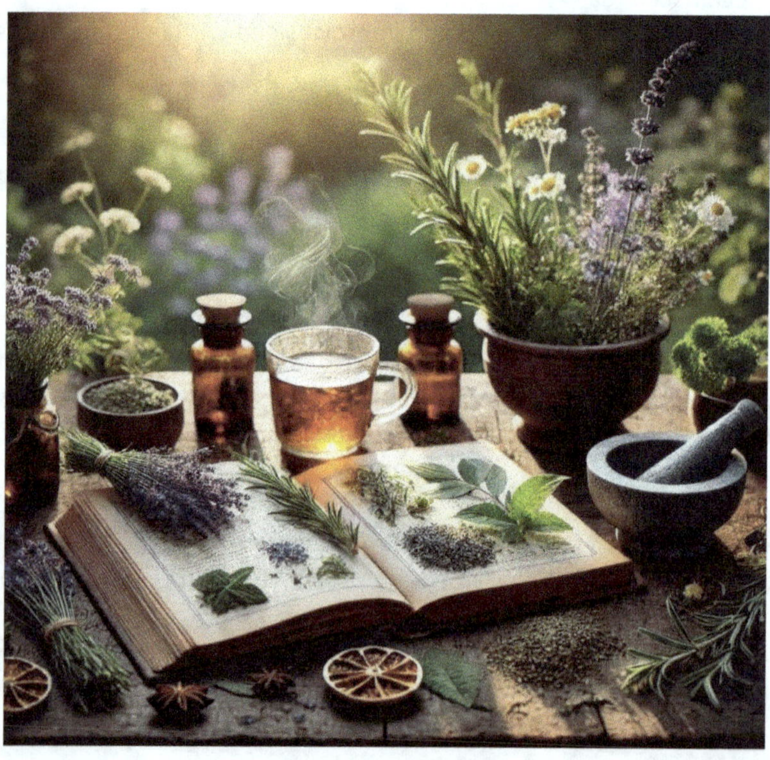

Chapter 1: Boosting Immunity

Recipe 1: Echinacea Immune-Boosting Tea

Deep within the vast prairies of North America, the indigenous peoples revered a humble flower for its healing prowess—the echinacea, or purple coneflower. This vibrant bloom was a cornerstone in traditional remedies, celebrated for enhancing the body's natural defenses. Today, echinacea remains a trusted ally in herbal medicine, offering a natural way to support and strengthen your immune system.

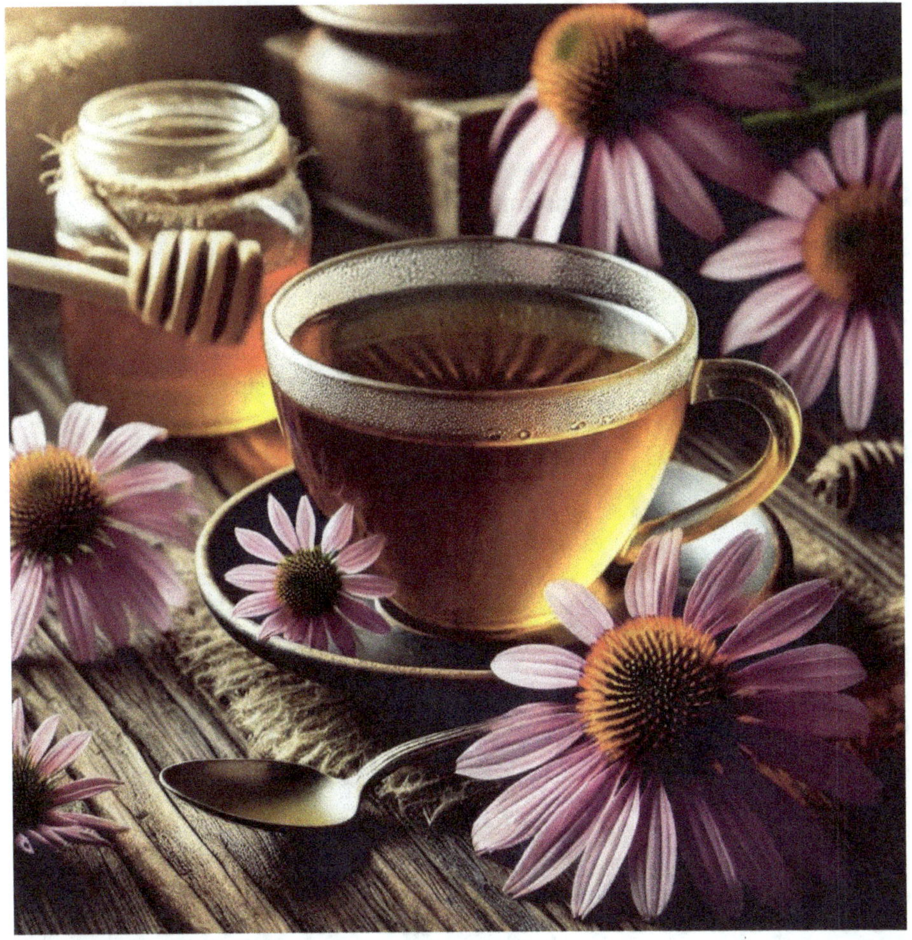

Ingredients:

- 1 tablespoon dried echinacea leaves and petals
- 1 teaspoon dried echinacea root (optional for added potency)

- 2 cups water
- Honey or lemon to taste

1. Bring the water to a boil in a small saucepan.
2. Add the dried echinacea leaves, petals, and root to the boiling water.
3. Reduce heat and let it simmer gently for 15 minutes.
4. Remove from heat and allow the tea to steep for an additional 5 minutes.
5. Strain the liquid into a mug.
6. Sweeten with honey or a squeeze of lemon if desired.

Usage:

Sip this nourishing tea up to three times daily, especially at the first sign of a cold or during times when your immune system needs extra support.

Caution:

If you have an autoimmune condition or are on immunosuppressant medications, consult a healthcare professional before using echinacea.

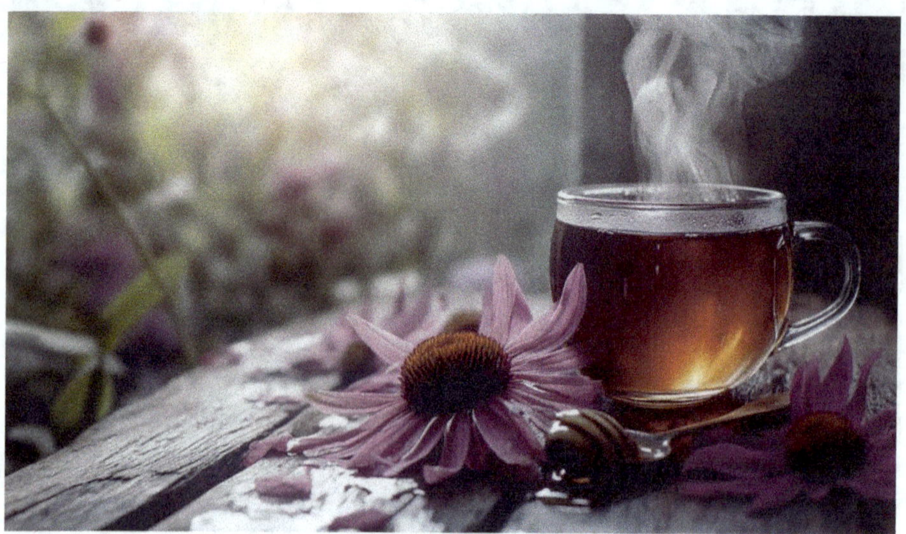

Recipe 2: Elderberry Syrup for Cold Prevention

In the folklore of Europe, elderberries were thought to possess magical properties, warding off evil and illness alike. Modern science has uncovered that these dark, glossy berries are rich in antioxidants and vitamins that may reduce the severity and duration of cold and flu symptoms. Crafting your own elderberry syrup is not only economical but also ensures you harness the full benefits of this potent berry.

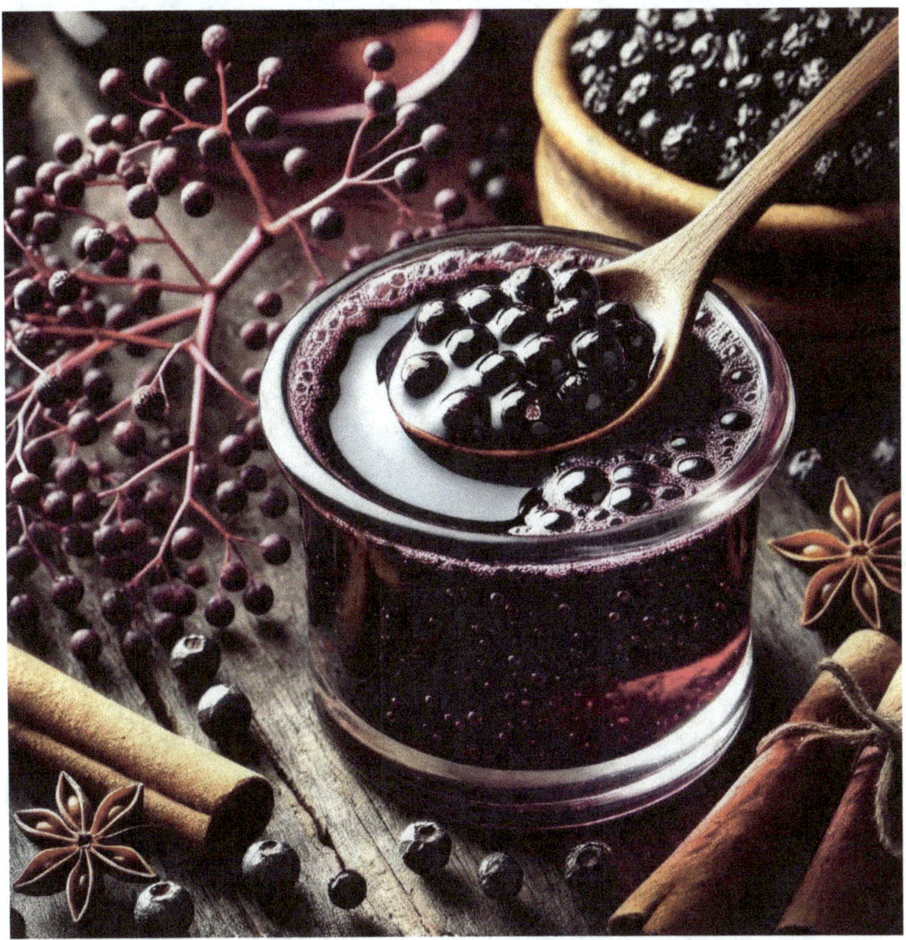

Ingredients:

- 1 cup fresh elderberries or ½ cup dried elderberries
- 4 cups water
- 1 cinnamon stick
- 1-inch piece fresh ginger, sliced

- 5 whole cloves
- 1 cup raw honey

Instructions:

1. In a medium saucepan, combine elderberries, water, cinnamon stick, ginger slices, and cloves.
2. Bring the mixture to a boil, then reduce the heat and simmer for about 45 minutes, until the liquid reduces by half.
3. Remove from heat and let it cool slightly.
4. Mash the berries thoroughly using a spoon or potato masher.
5. Strain the mixture through a fine mesh strainer or cheesecloth into a bowl, pressing down to extract all the liquid.
6. Add raw honey to the warm liquid and stir well until fully dissolved.
7. Transfer the syrup to a sterilized glass jar with a lid and store it in the refrigerator.

Usage:

Take 1 tablespoon daily for adults and 1 teaspoon daily for children over one year old as a preventive measure. During illness, take the same dosage every 2-3 hours until symptoms improve.

Caution:

Ensure elderberries are fully cooked, as raw elderberries can be toxic. Do not give honey to children under one year of age.

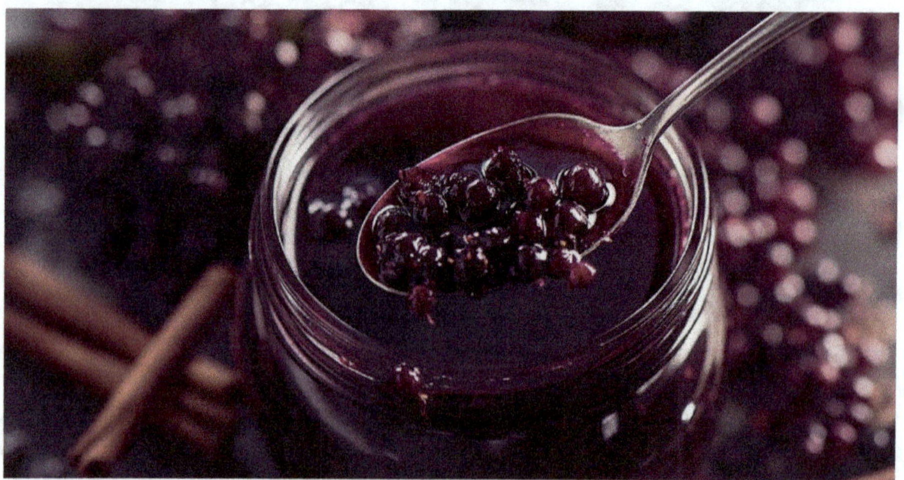

Recipe 3: Garlic and Honey Elixir for Fighting Infections

Garlic, with its pungent aroma and robust flavor, has been a medicinal staple across cultures for millennia. Ancient civilizations used it not just for culinary purposes but as a powerful remedy for various ailments. When combined with the natural soothing properties of honey, garlic transforms into a formidable elixir that can help fend off infections and boost overall health.

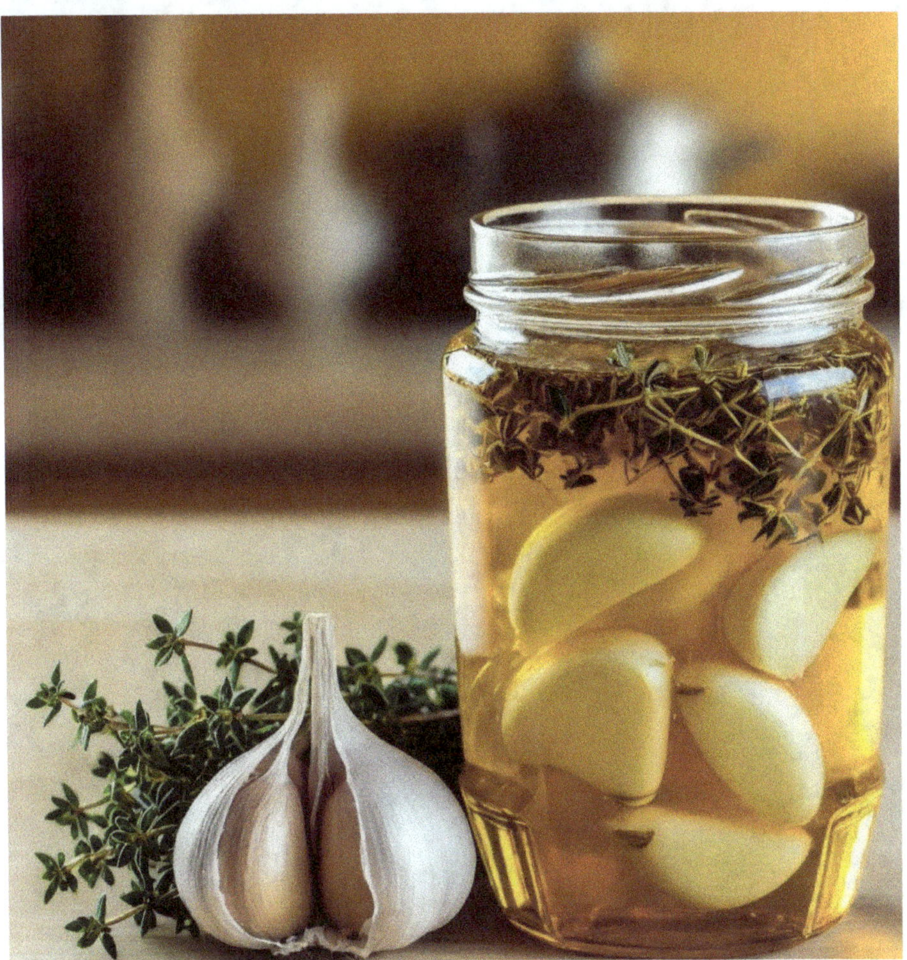

Ingredients:

- 1 cup raw honey
- 10 cloves fresh garlic, peeled and lightly crushed
- Optional: A few sprigs of fresh thyme or a pinch of dried thyme

Instructions:

1. Place the crushed garlic cloves (and thyme, if using) into a clean, dry glass jar.
2. Pour the raw honey over the garlic, ensuring all cloves are fully submerged.
3. Seal the jar tightly with a lid.
4. Allow the mixture to infuse at room temperature for at least 5 days. The honey will become thinner as the garlic releases its juices.
5. Gently turn the jar upside down daily to mix the contents.

Usage:

At the onset of a cold or infection, take 1 teaspoon of the elixir every few hours. For general immune support, consume 1 teaspoon daily.

Caution:

Garlic may interact with certain medications, such as anticoagulants. Consult a healthcare provider if you are on medication or have a bleeding disorder.

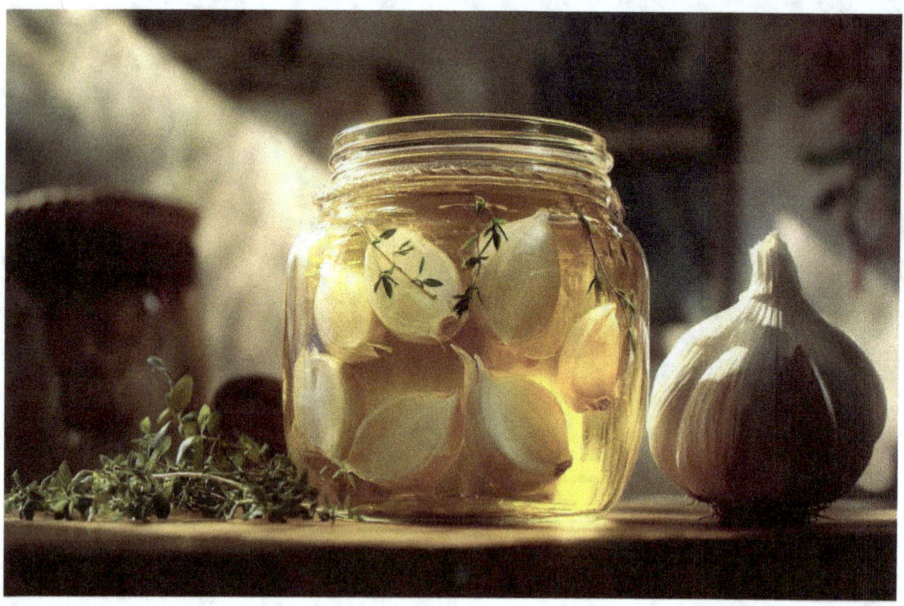

Recipe 4: Turmeric Golden Milk for Inflammation

Golden milk, a traditional Ayurvedic beverage, has been cherished in India for centuries. The star ingredient, turmeric, is renowned for its anti-inflammatory and antioxidant properties, largely due to the compound curcumin. This warm, soothing drink not only comforts the soul but also supports joint health and overall wellness.

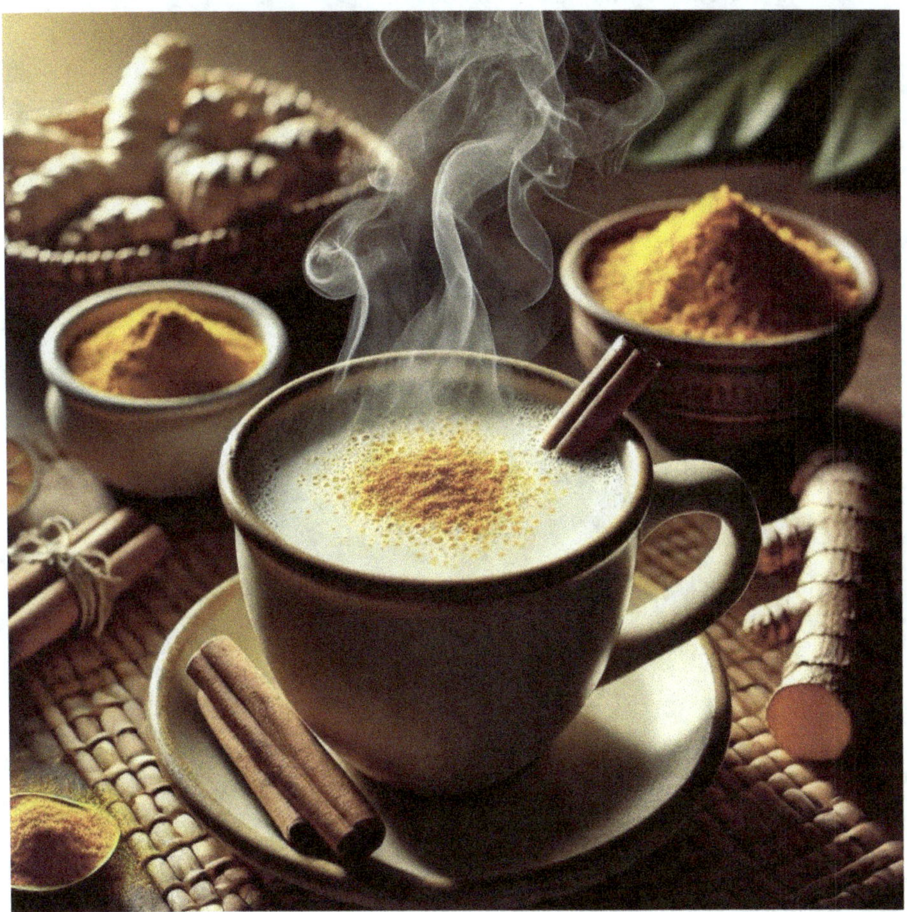

Ingredients:

- 1 cup milk of your choice (dairy, almond, coconut, etc.)
- 1 teaspoon ground turmeric
- ¼ teaspoon ground cinnamon
- Pinch of black pepper (enhances turmeric absorption)
- ½ teaspoon raw honey or maple syrup (optional, for sweetness)
- Small piece of fresh ginger, grated (optional)

Instructions:

1. In a small saucepan, combine all ingredients except the sweetener.
2. Heat over medium heat until the mixture is hot but not boiling, stirring continuously.
3. Reduce heat and simmer for 5 minutes to allow the flavors to meld.
4. Remove from heat and strain if using fresh ginger.
5. Stir in honey or maple syrup if desired.
6. Pour into a mug and enjoy warm.

Usage:

Drink once daily, preferably in the evening, to promote relaxation and reduce inflammation.

Caution:

Consult your doctor if you are taking medication for blood thinning or gallbladder issues, as turmeric can have contraindications.

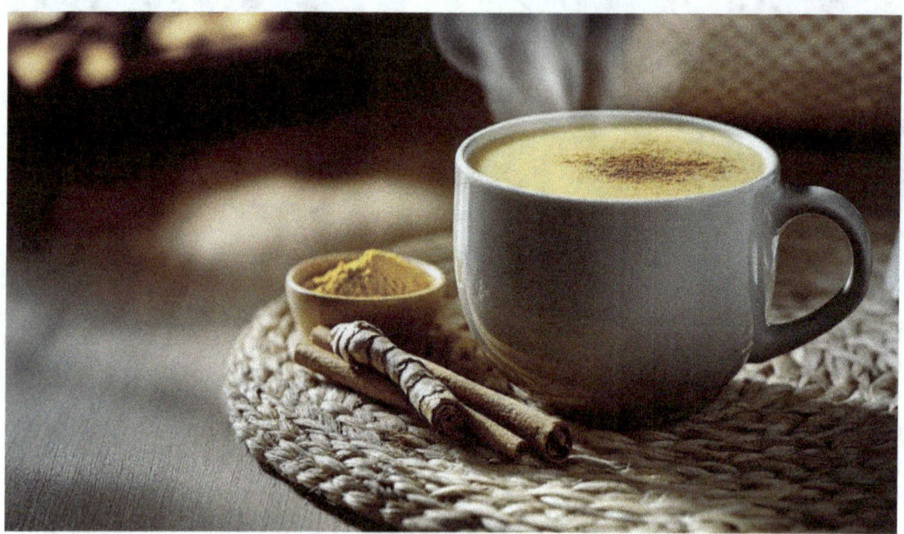

Recipe 5: Astragalus Root Soup for Strengthening Defenses

Astragalus root, a staple in Traditional Chinese Medicine, is esteemed for its ability to strengthen Qi—the body's vital energy. This adaptogenic herb is known to enhance resilience against stress and bolster the immune system. Incorporating astragalus into a nourishing soup makes for a delicious way to fortify your body's defenses.

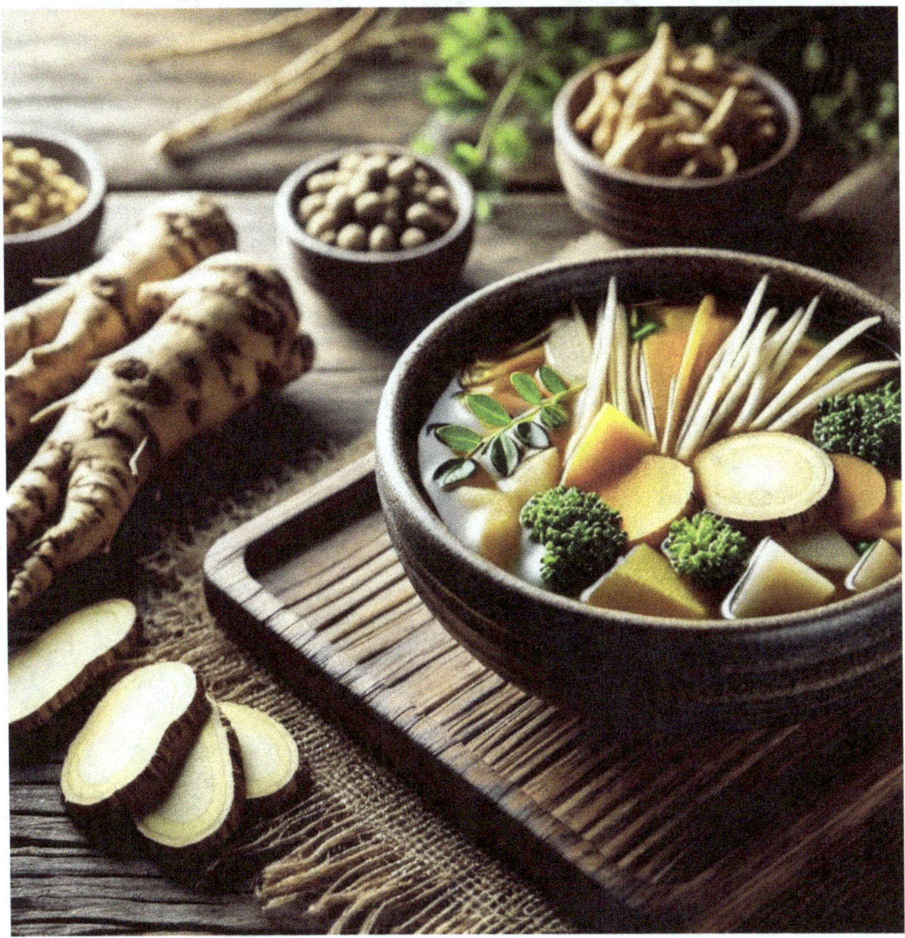

Ingredients:

- 3-4 slices of dried astragalus root
- 8 cups vegetable or chicken broth
- 1 onion, chopped
- 2 carrots, sliced
- 2 celery stalks, chopped

- 2 cloves garlic, minced
- 1 cup sliced mushrooms (optional)
- Salt and pepper to taste
- Fresh parsley or cilantro for garnish

Instructions:

1. In a large pot, sauté onions, carrots, and celery over medium heat until softened.
2. Add minced garlic and cook for an additional minute.
3. Pour in the broth and add the astragalus root slices and mushrooms if using.
4. Bring the soup to a boil, then reduce heat and simmer for 30-45 minutes.
5. Remove the astragalus root slices before serving.
6. Season with salt and pepper to taste.
7. Ladle into bowls and garnish with fresh parsley or cilantro.

Usage:

Enjoy this soup regularly during the colder months or whenever your immune system needs a boost.

Caution:

Astragalus may interact with immunosuppressive drugs. Consult a healthcare professional if you are on such medications.

Note: These recipes are meant to support general wellness and are not a substitute for professional medical advice. Always consult with a healthcare provider before starting any new health regimen, especially if you have underlying health conditions or are pregnant or nursing.

Recipe 6: Ginger Digestive Aid Tea

For millennia, ginger has been a cornerstone in traditional medicine across Asia and beyond. Revered for its warming properties and distinctive spicy flavor, ginger is celebrated for its ability to soothe an upset stomach, alleviate nausea, and promote healthy digestion. A simple ginger tea can be a comforting companion after a heavy meal or during times of digestive discomfort.

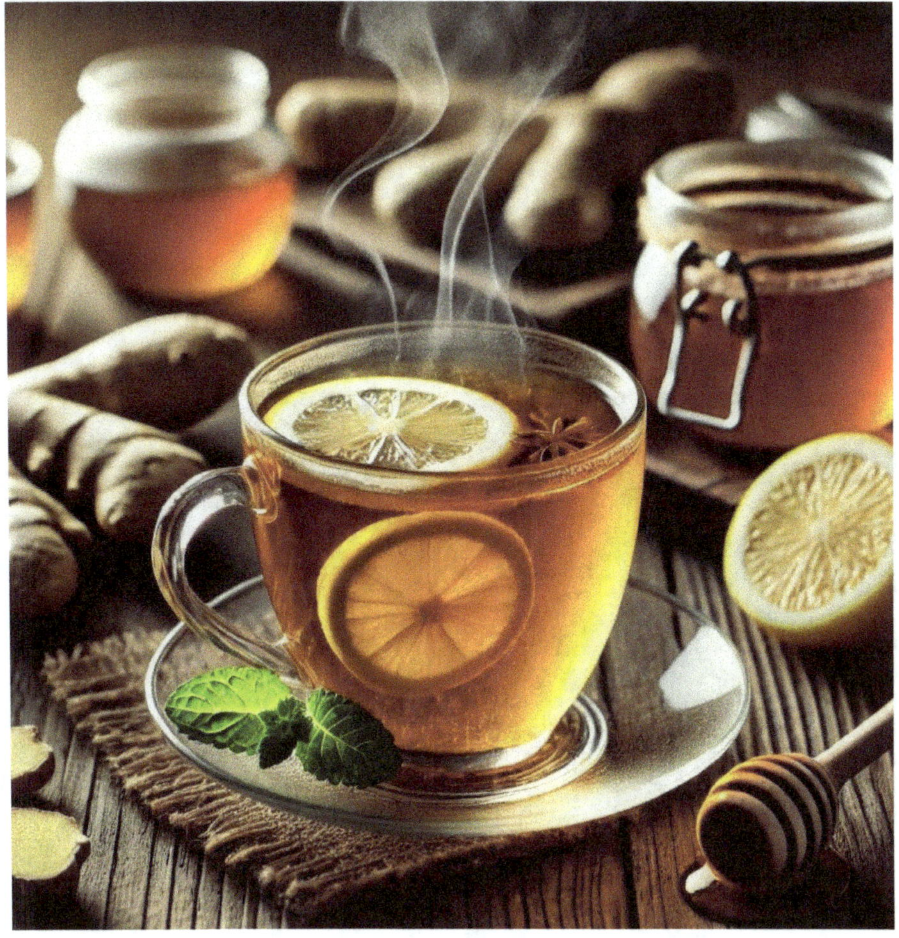

Ingredients:

- 1-inch piece of fresh ginger root, thinly sliced or grated
- 2 cups water

- Juice of half a lemon (optional)
- Honey or maple syrup to taste (optional)

Instructions:

1. Bring the water to a boil in a small saucepan.
2. Add the sliced or grated ginger to the boiling water.
3. Reduce heat and let it simmer for 10–15 minutes.
4. Remove from heat and strain the tea into a mug.
5. Stir in lemon juice and honey or maple syrup if desired.
6. Sip slowly and enjoy the soothing warmth.

Usage:

Drink this tea after meals to aid digestion or whenever you experience nausea or stomach discomfort.

Caution:

Consult a healthcare professional if you are taking blood-thinning medications or have gallstones.

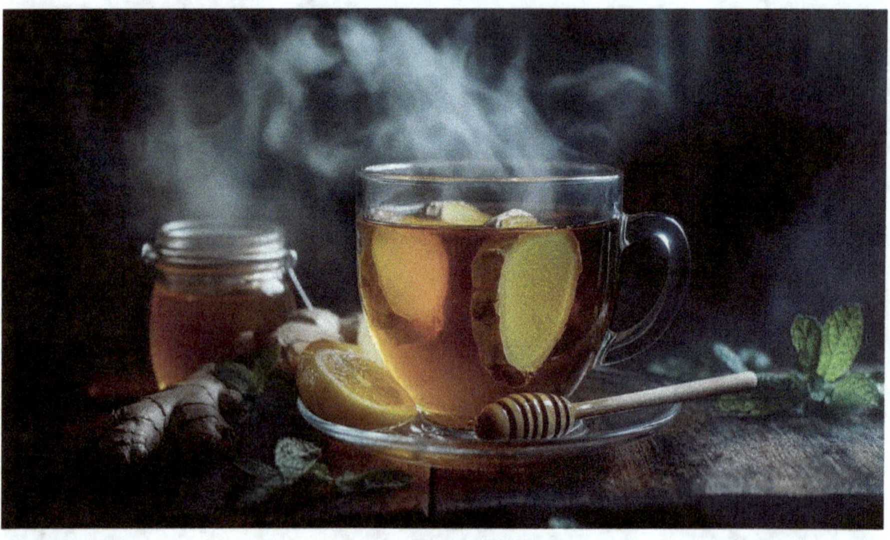

Recipe 7: Peppermint Infusion for Indigestion Relief

Peppermint, with its refreshing aroma and cool taste, has been used since ancient times to ease digestive woes. Its natural compounds help relax the stomach muscles and improve the flow of bile, making it an effective remedy for indigestion, gas, and bloating. A cup of peppermint tea can bring swift relief and a moment of tranquility.

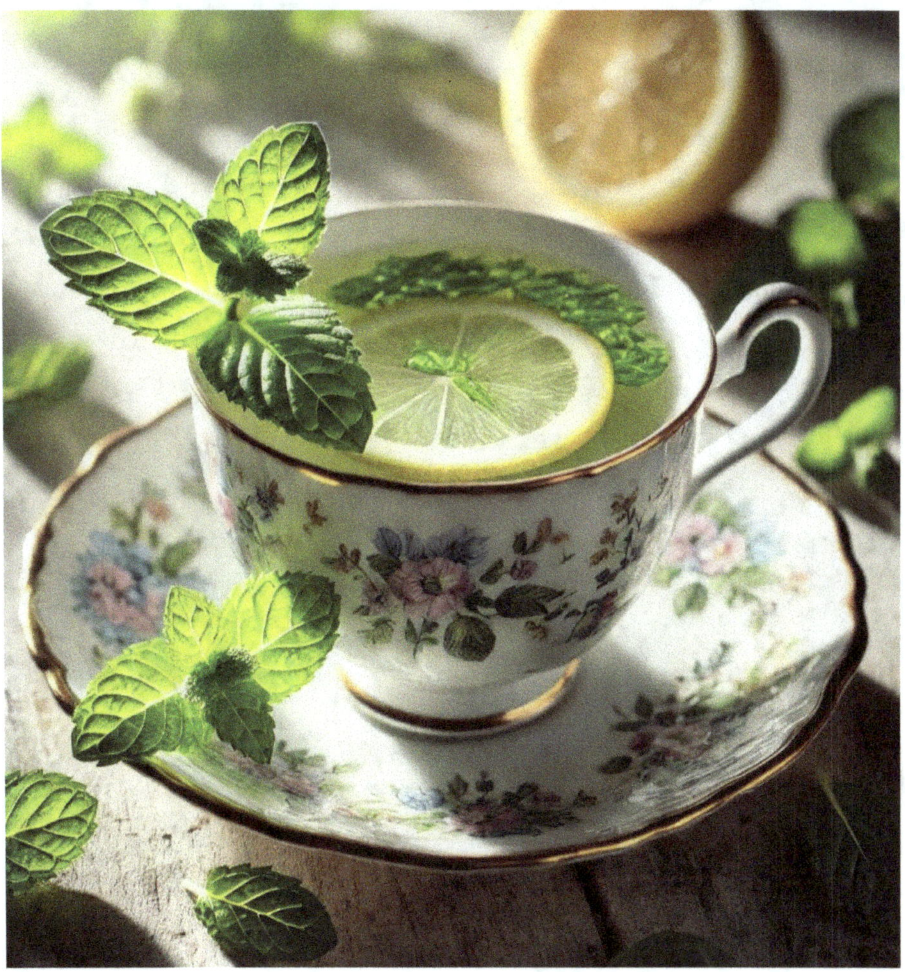

Ingredients:

- 1 teaspoon dried peppermint leaves or a handful of fresh leaves
- 1 cup boiling water
- Honey or lemon to taste (optional)

1. Place the peppermint leaves in a teapot or directly into your cup.
2. Pour boiling water over the leaves.
3. Cover and let steep for 5–7 minutes.
4. Strain the tea into a cup if brewed loose.
5. Add honey or lemon if desired for additional flavor.
6. Enjoy warm.

Enjoy a cup after meals or whenever you feel digestive discomfort.

Not recommended for individuals with gastroesophageal reflux disease (GERD), as peppermint may exacerbate symptoms.

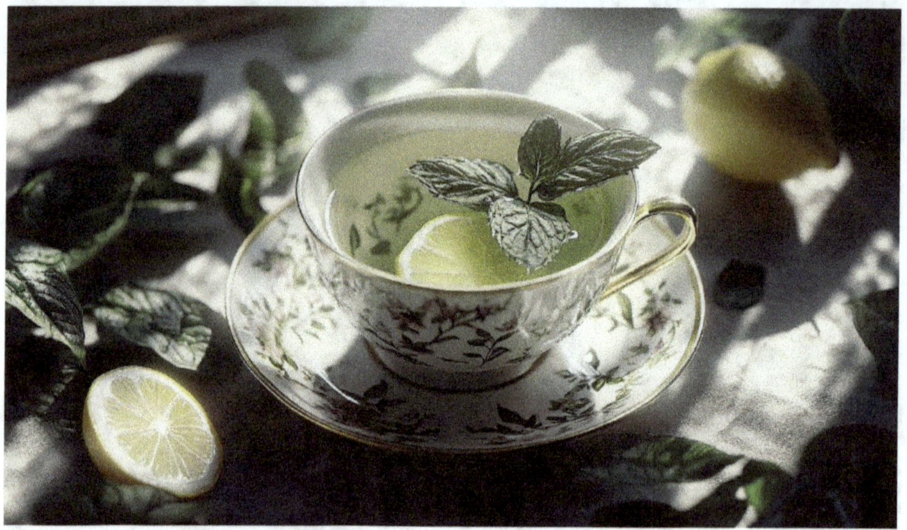

Recipe 8: Fennel Seed Chew for Bloating

In various cultures, particularly in India, chewing fennel seeds after a meal is a common practice to aid digestion and freshen breath. Fennel seeds possess carminative properties, helping to reduce gas, bloating, and stomach cramps. Their sweet, anise-like flavor makes them a pleasant natural remedy.

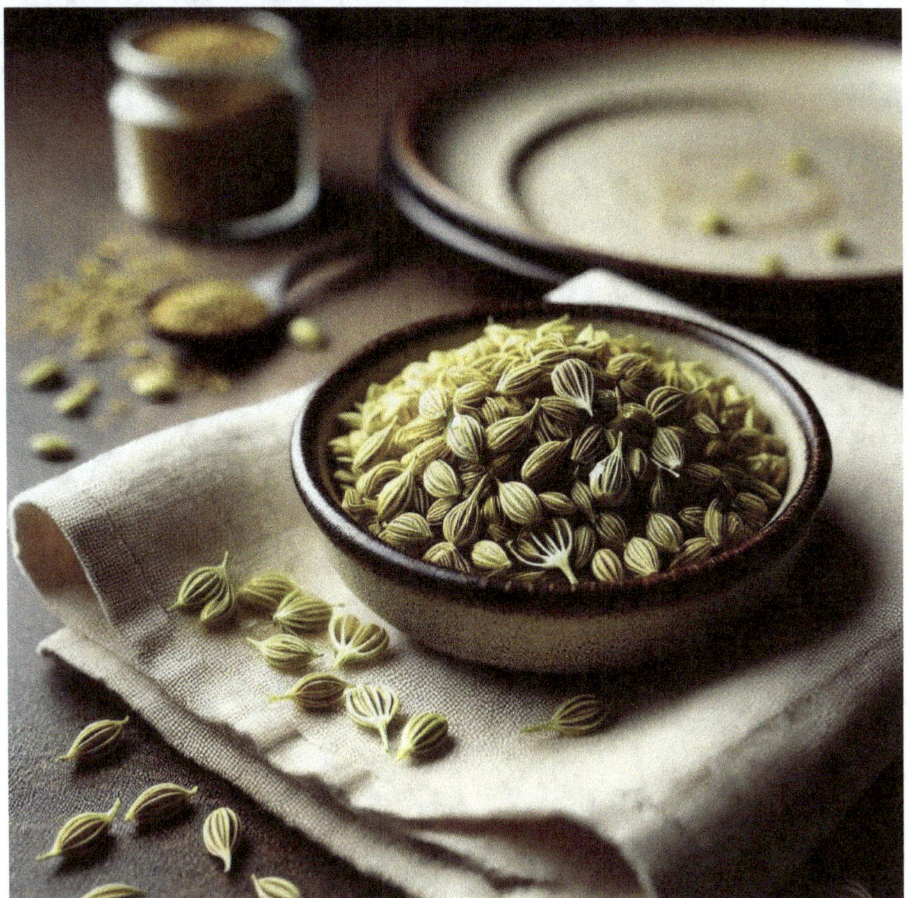

Ingredients:

- 1 teaspoon fennel seeds

Instructions:

1. Measure out a teaspoon of fennel seeds.
2. Chew the seeds thoroughly after your meal.
3. Swallow after chewing to ingest the beneficial oils.

Use after meals to promote digestion and alleviate bloating.

While fennel is generally safe, those with allergies to celery, carrot, or mugwort may also react to fennel.

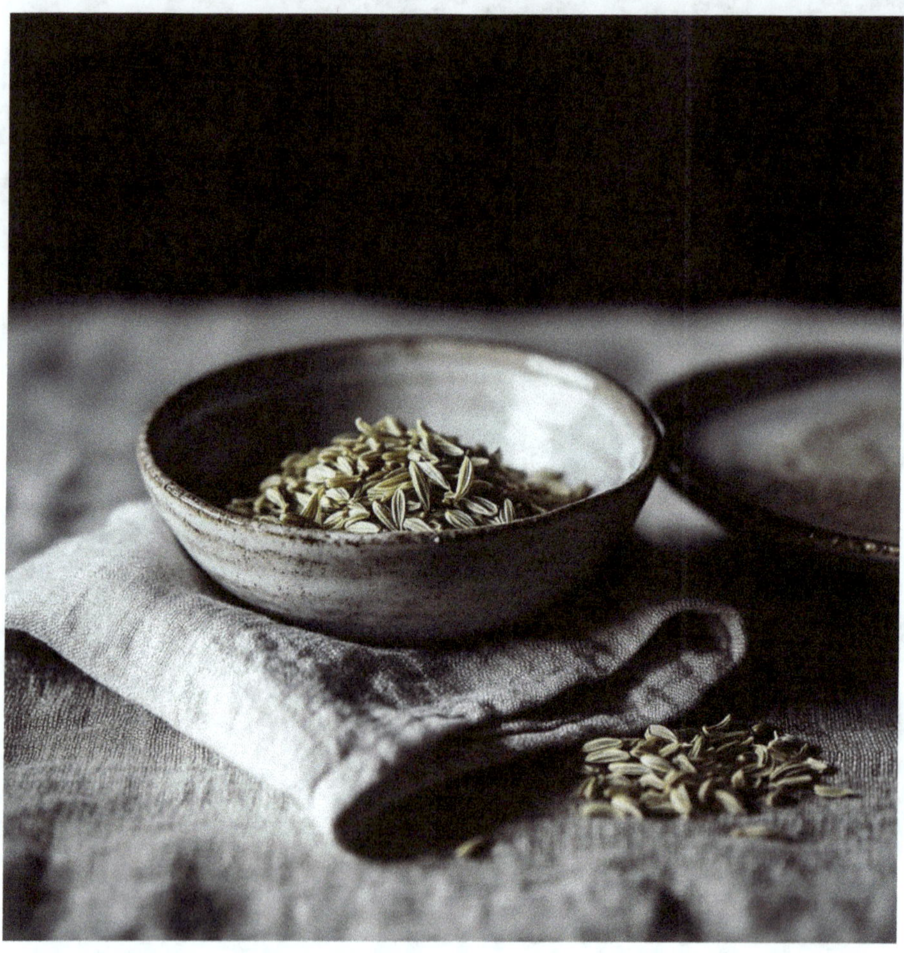

Recipe 9: Chamomile and Licorice Soothing Tea

Chamomile is renowned for its gentle calming effects, both on the nervous and digestive systems. When combined with licorice root, which has anti-inflammatory and mucosal-protective properties, this tea becomes a powerful ally against indigestion, heartburn, and stomach ulcers. The blend offers a sweet, soothing flavor that comforts both body and mind.

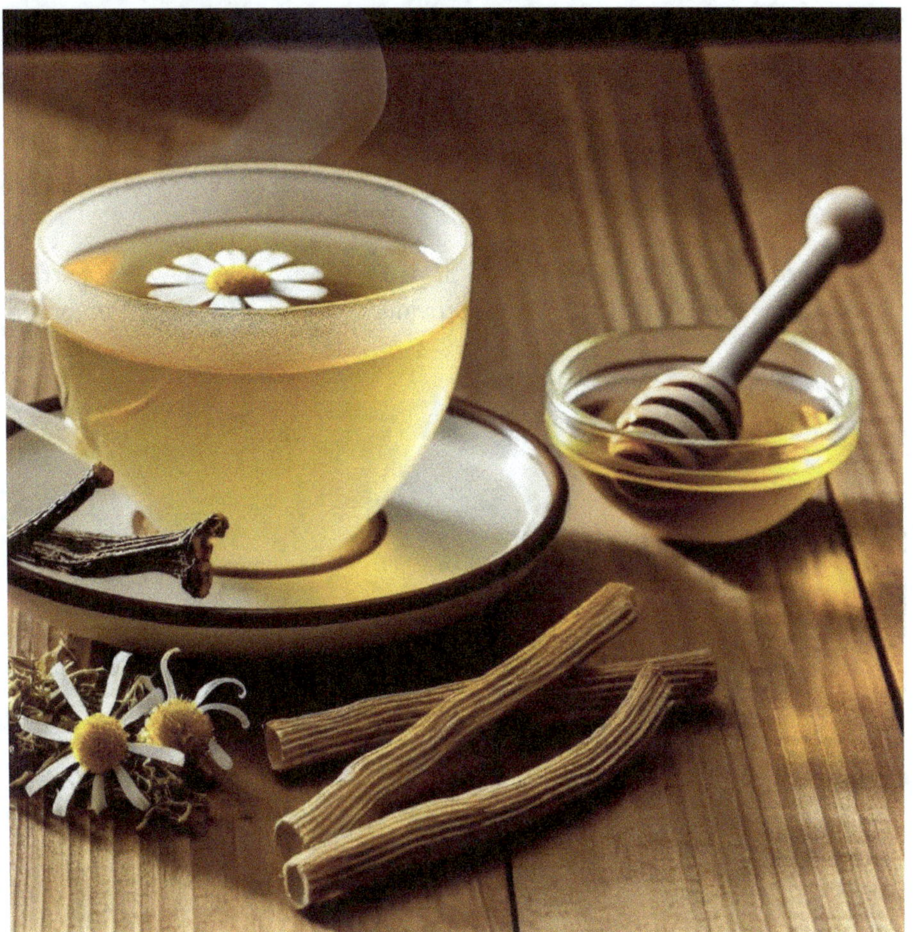

Ingredients:

- 2 teaspoons dried chamomile flowers
- 1 teaspoon dried licorice root
- 1 cup boiling water
- Honey to taste (optional)

1. Combine chamomile flowers and licorice root in a teapot or infuser.
2. Pour boiling water over the herbs.
3. Cover and let steep for 10 minutes to extract the full benefits.
4. Strain the tea into a cup.
5. Add honey if desired for added sweetness.
6. Enjoy while warm, savoring each sip.

Usage:

Drink up to twice daily to soothe digestive discomfort.

Caution:

Licorice root may elevate blood pressure and interact with certain medications. Consult your healthcare provider if you have hypertension or are on medication.

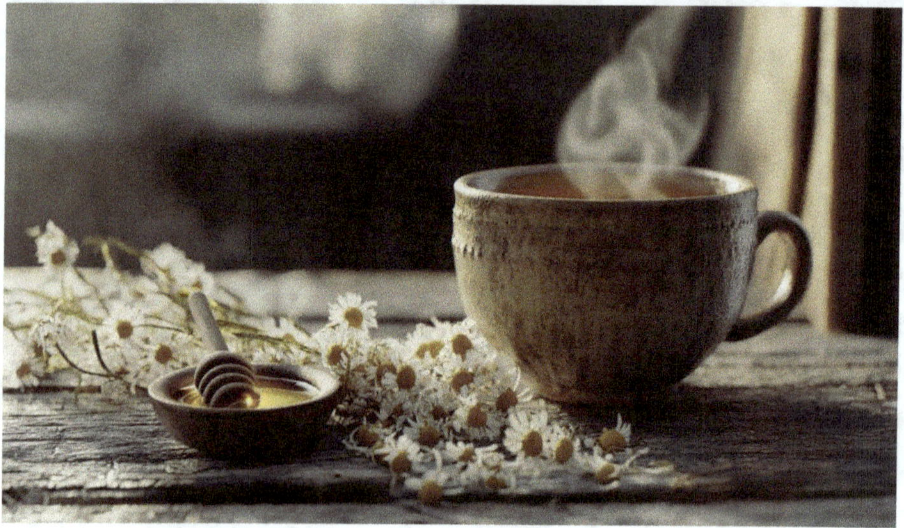

Recipe 10: Dandelion Root Coffee Alternative for Liver Health

Dandelion roots have been used for centuries to support liver and digestive health. When roasted, they offer a rich, coffee-like flavor without the caffeine, making them an excellent substitute for traditional coffee. This brew not only satisfies your taste buds but also promotes bile production, aiding in the digestion of fats and the elimination of toxins.

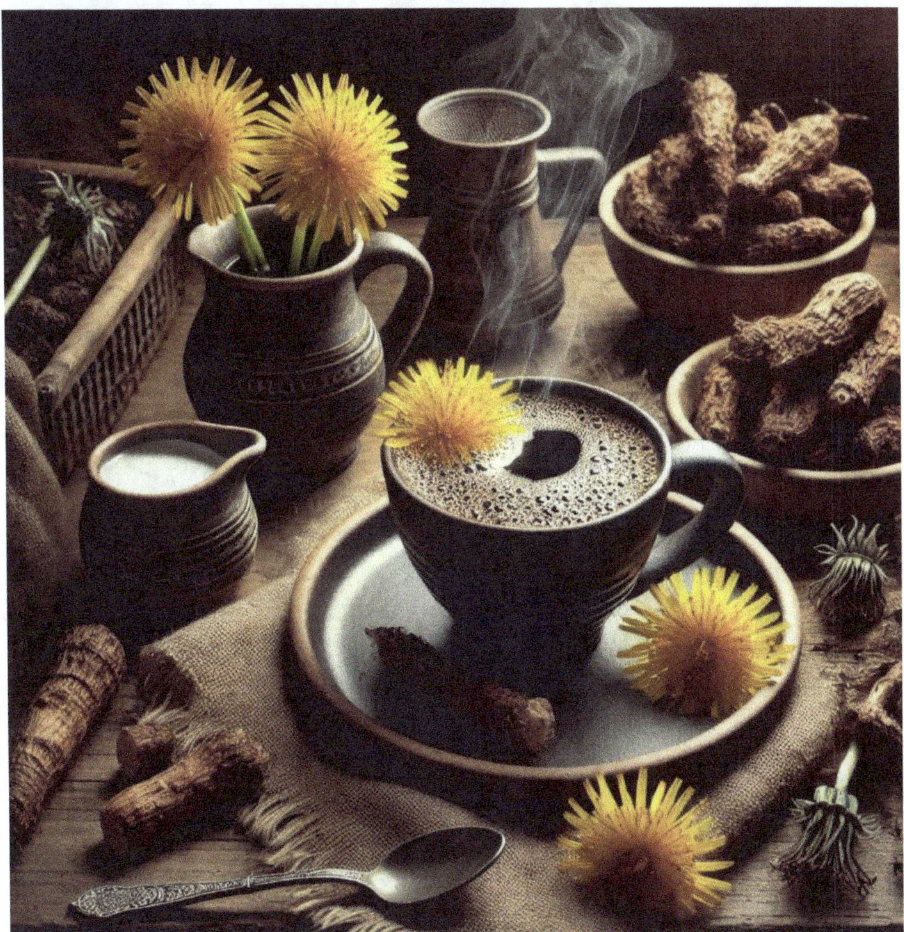

Ingredients:

- 2 teaspoons roasted dandelion root granules
- 1 cup water
- Milk or dairy alternative (optional)
- Sweetener of choice (optional)

1. Place roasted dandelion root in a small saucepan with water.
2. Bring to a gentle boil, then reduce heat and simmer for 5–10 minutes.
3. Strain the liquid into a mug.
4. Add milk and sweetener if desired, stirring well.
5. Enjoy hot, savoring the rich flavor.

Usage:

Replace your regular coffee with this dandelion brew to support digestion and liver function.

Caution:

Avoid if you have gallstones or bile duct obstruction. Consult a healthcare professional if you are on medication, as dandelion may interact with certain drugs.

Note: The recipes provided are for general wellness and informational purposes. They are not intended to diagnose, treat, cure, or prevent any disease. Please consult a healthcare professional before incorporating new remedies into your routine, especially if you have existing health conditions, are pregnant, or are breastfeeding.

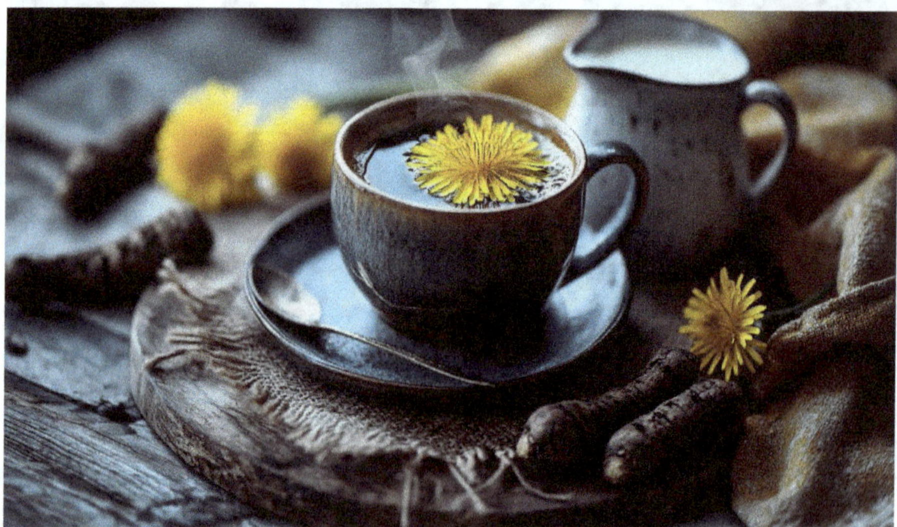

Recipe 11: Lavender Calming Bath Soak

Lavender, with its delicate purple blossoms and enchanting scent, has been a symbol of serenity and calm for centuries. The ancient Egyptians used it in perfumes, while the Romans infused their bathwater with lavender to unwind after battles. Today, this aromatic herb remains a beloved remedy for stress and sleeplessness. A lavender-infused bath soak is a luxurious way to ease tension and prepare your mind and body for restful slumber.

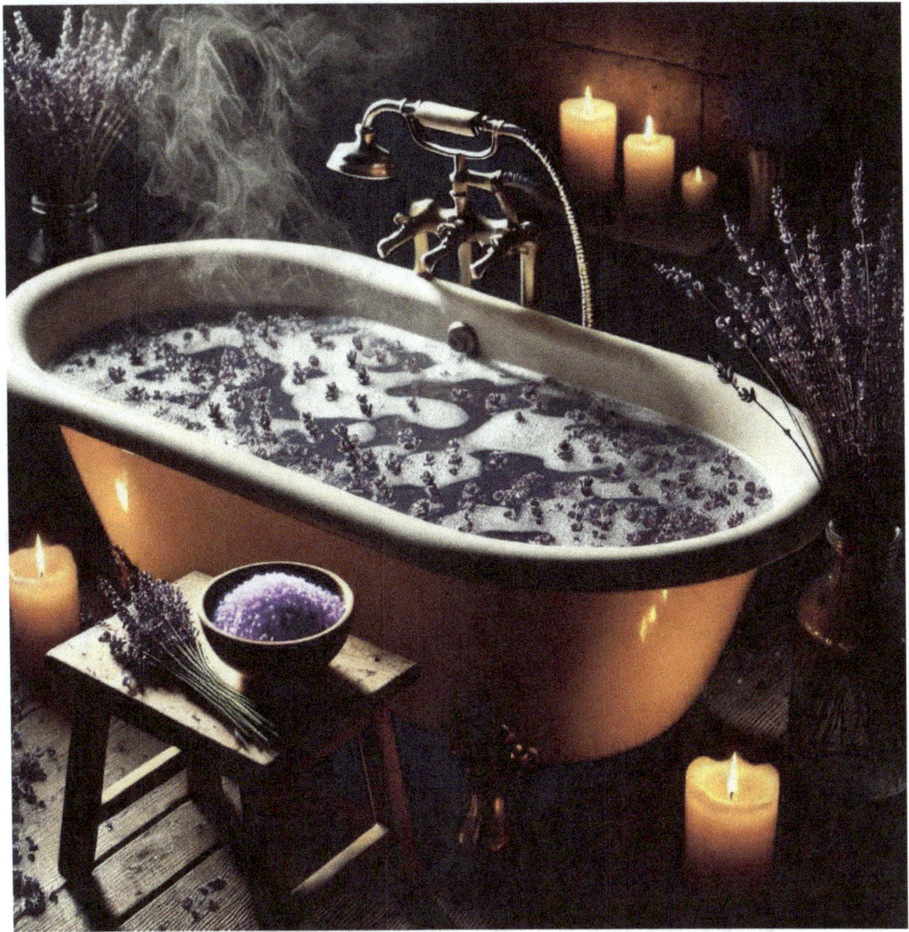

Ingredients:

- 1 cup Epsom salts
- ½ cup dried lavender flowers

- 10 drops lavender essential oil
- ¼ cup baking soda (optional, for skin softening)
- Muslin bag or cheesecloth (optional, to contain the herbs)

Instructions:

1. In a mixing bowl, combine Epsom salts and baking soda.
2. Stir in the dried lavender flowers.
3. Add the lavender essential oil, mixing thoroughly to distribute the scent evenly.
4. If using a muslin bag or cheesecloth, fill it with the mixture and tie securely.
5. Fill your bathtub with warm water.
6. Add the lavender bath soak directly to the water or hang the filled muslin bag under the faucet as the tub fills.
7. Soak in the bath for at least 20 minutes, breathing deeply to inhale the calming aroma.

Usage:

Enjoy this relaxing bath in the evening to help unwind after a stressful day and promote a good night's sleep.

Caution:

- Be cautious when exiting the tub, as the oils may make surfaces slippery.
- If pregnant or breastfeeding, consult a healthcare professional before using essential oils.
- Discontinue use if skin irritation occurs.

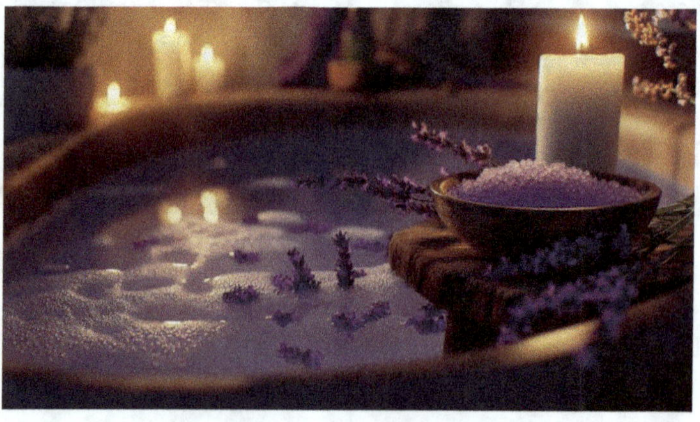

Recipe 12: Valerian Root Sleep Tincture

Valerian root, often referred to as "nature's Valium," has a long history as a gentle sedative and sleep aid. Used since ancient Greek and Roman times, valerian is known for its ability to improve sleep quality without the grogginess associated with some medications. Creating a tincture allows you to harness the full potency of valerian root in a convenient form.

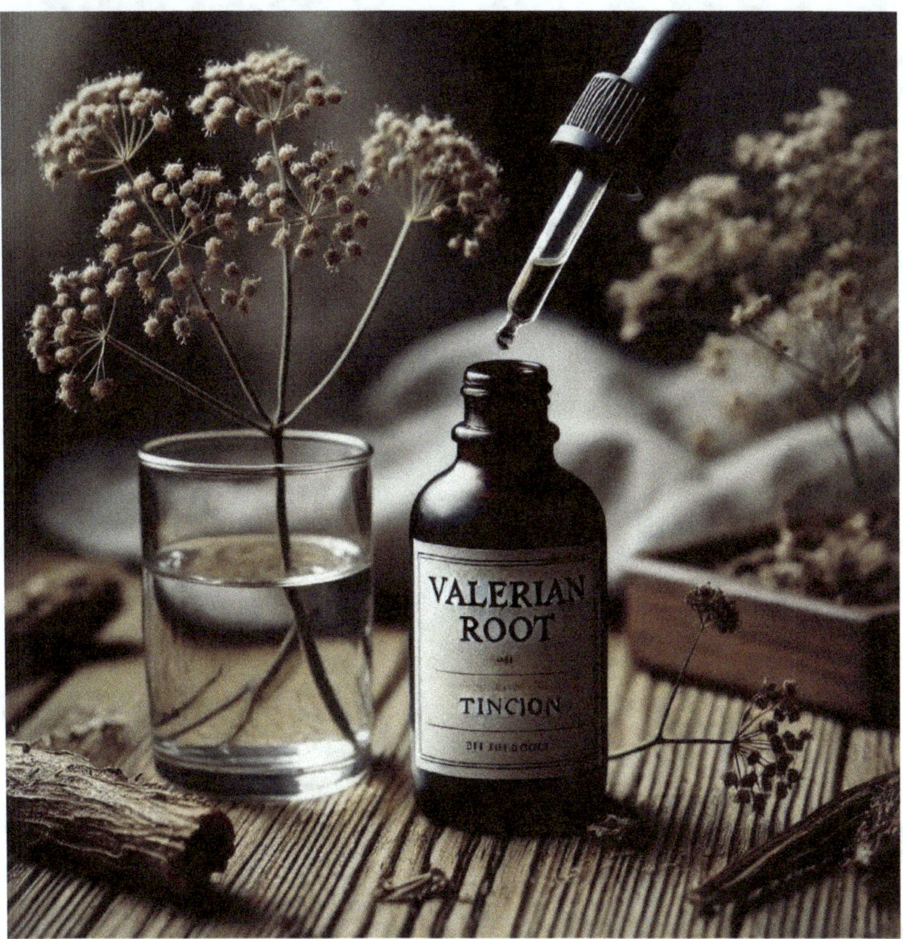

Ingredients:

- 1 cup dried valerian root
- 2 cups vodka or glycerin (for an alcohol-free option)
- A clean glass jar with a tight-fitting lid
- Dark glass dropper bottles for storage

1. Place the dried valerian root into the glass jar.
2. Pour vodka or glycerin over the root until completely covered, leaving about an inch of liquid above the herbs.
3. Seal the jar tightly and shake well.
4. Store the jar in a cool, dark place for 4–6 weeks, shaking it daily to mix the contents.
5. After steeping, strain the liquid through a fine mesh strainer or cheesecloth into a clean bowl, pressing the root to extract as much liquid as possible.
6. Transfer the tincture into dark glass dropper bottles for storage.
7. Label the bottles with the contents and date.

Usage:

Take 1–2 droppers full (approximately 30–60 drops) in a small amount of water or juice about 30 minutes before bedtime.

Caution:

- Valerian may cause drowsiness; do not drive or operate heavy machinery after taking.
- Not recommended for use during pregnancy or breastfeeding.
- Consult a healthcare provider if you are taking other sedatives or medications.

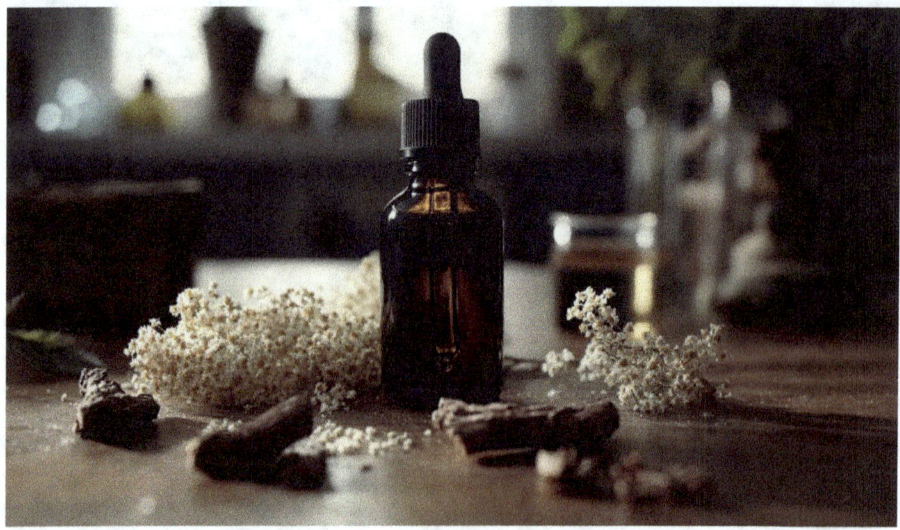

Recipe 13: Passionflower Tea for Anxiety Reduction

Native to the southeastern United States, passionflower was traditionally used by Native Americans for its calming properties. The intricate, exotic blossoms of passionflower are as soothing to the mind as they are beautiful to the eye. This gentle herb is effective in reducing anxiety and promoting restful sleep, making it a valuable addition to your relaxation routine.

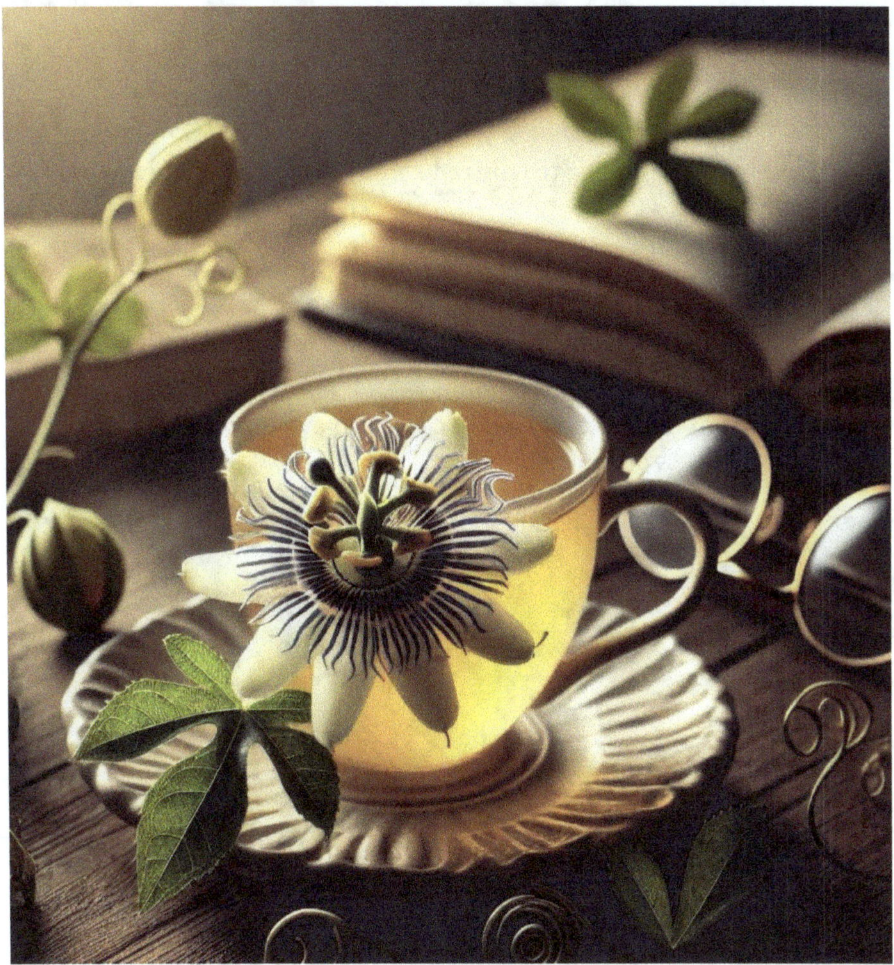

Ingredients:

- 1 teaspoon dried passionflower herb
- 1 cup boiling water
- Honey or lemon to taste (optional)

1. Place the dried passionflower in a tea infuser or teapot.
2. Pour boiling water over the herb.
3. Cover and let steep for 10 minutes to extract the beneficial compounds.
4. Strain the tea into a cup.
5. Add honey or lemon if desired.
6. Sip slowly, focusing on relaxation.

Usage:

Drink one cup in the evening to help reduce anxiety and promote sleep.

Caution:

- Not recommended for pregnant or breastfeeding women.
- May interact with sedatives or anti-anxiety medications; consult a healthcare professional before use.
- Do not exceed recommended dosage to avoid potential side effects like dizziness or confusion.

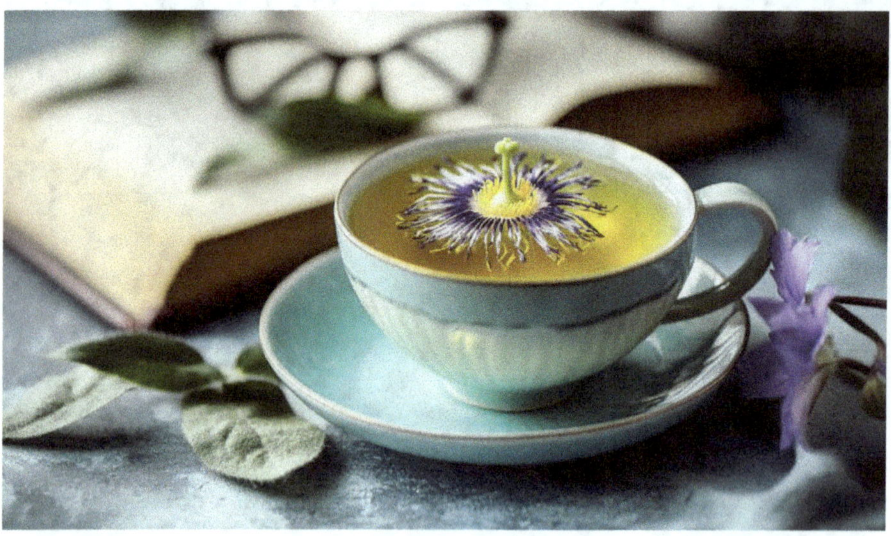

Recipe 14: Lemon Balm Relaxation Elixir

Lemon balm, a member of the mint family, exudes a delightful citrus scent that has been used since the Middle Ages to reduce stress and anxiety, promote sleep, and improve digestion. Known as the "gladdening herb," lemon balm lifts the spirits while calming the nerves. This simple elixir is a pleasant way to unwind and enhance your mood.

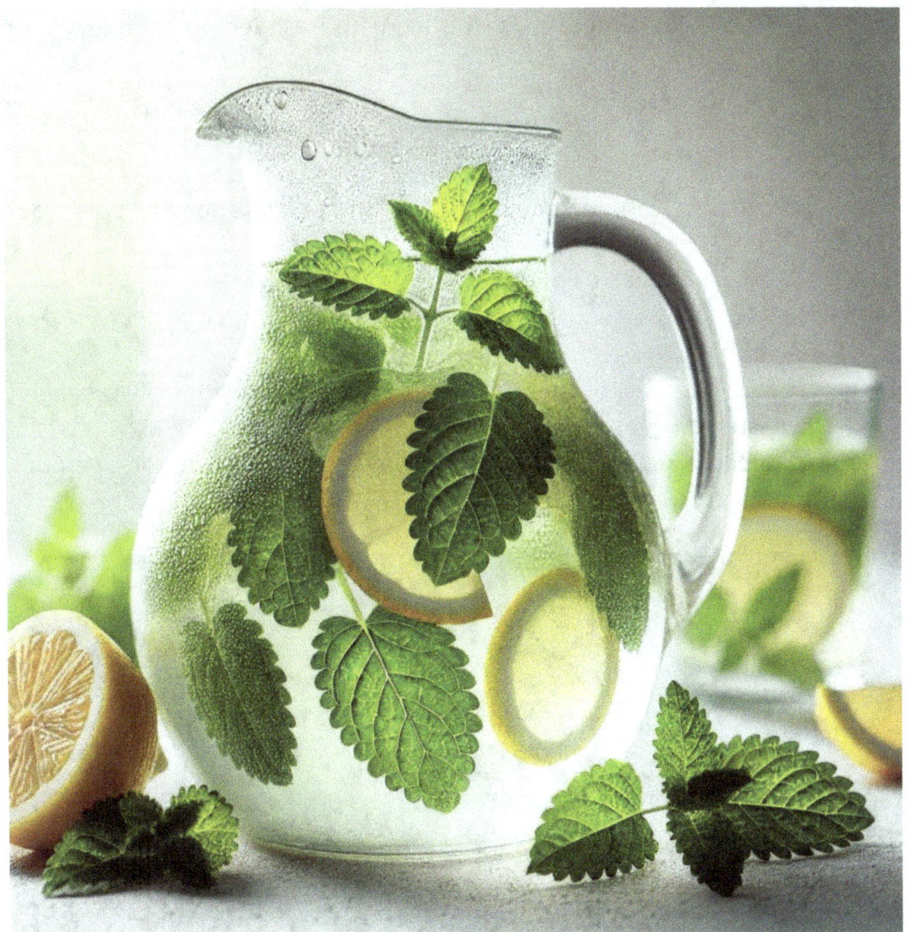

Ingredients:

- 1 cup fresh lemon balm leaves (or ½ cup dried)
- 4 cups water
- Juice of one lemon
- Honey or agave syrup to taste
- Ice cubes (optional)

1. In a saucepan, bring the water to a boil.
2. Remove from heat and add the lemon balm leaves.
3. Cover and let steep for 15 minutes.
4. Strain the liquid into a pitcher.
5. Stir in the lemon juice and sweeten with honey or agave syrup to taste.
6. Allow the elixir to cool to room temperature or refrigerate.
7. Serve over ice if desired, garnished with fresh lemon balm leaves or lemon slices.

Usage:

Enjoy a glass in the afternoon or evening to promote relaxation and uplift your mood.

Caution:

- Generally safe, but consult a healthcare provider if pregnant, breastfeeding, or taking thyroid medications.
- May cause drowsiness; exercise caution when driving or operating machinery.

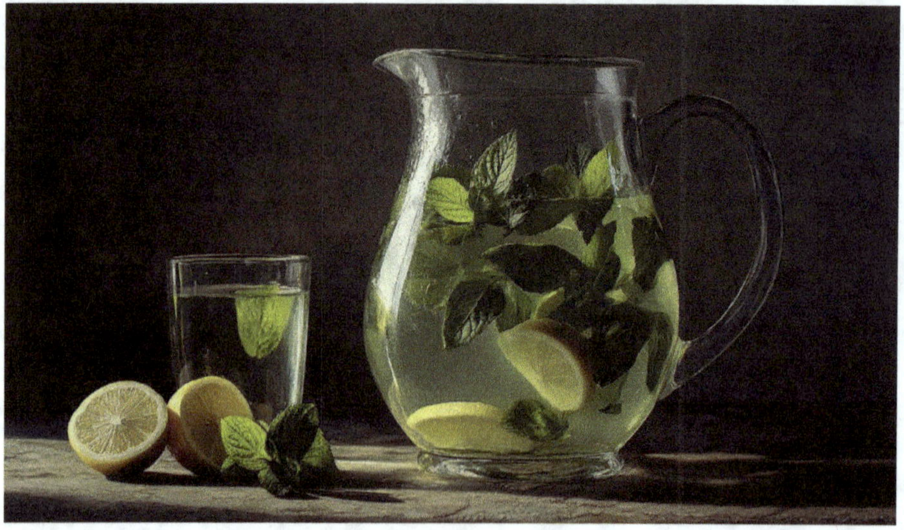

Recipe 15: Hops Pillow Sachets for Restful Sleep

Hops are best known for their role in brewing beer, but these cone-shaped flowers have also been used traditionally to promote sleep and relieve restlessness. The sedative properties of hops make them an excellent natural remedy for insomnia. Creating a hops-infused pillow sachet allows you to benefit from their calming effects aromatically throughout the night.

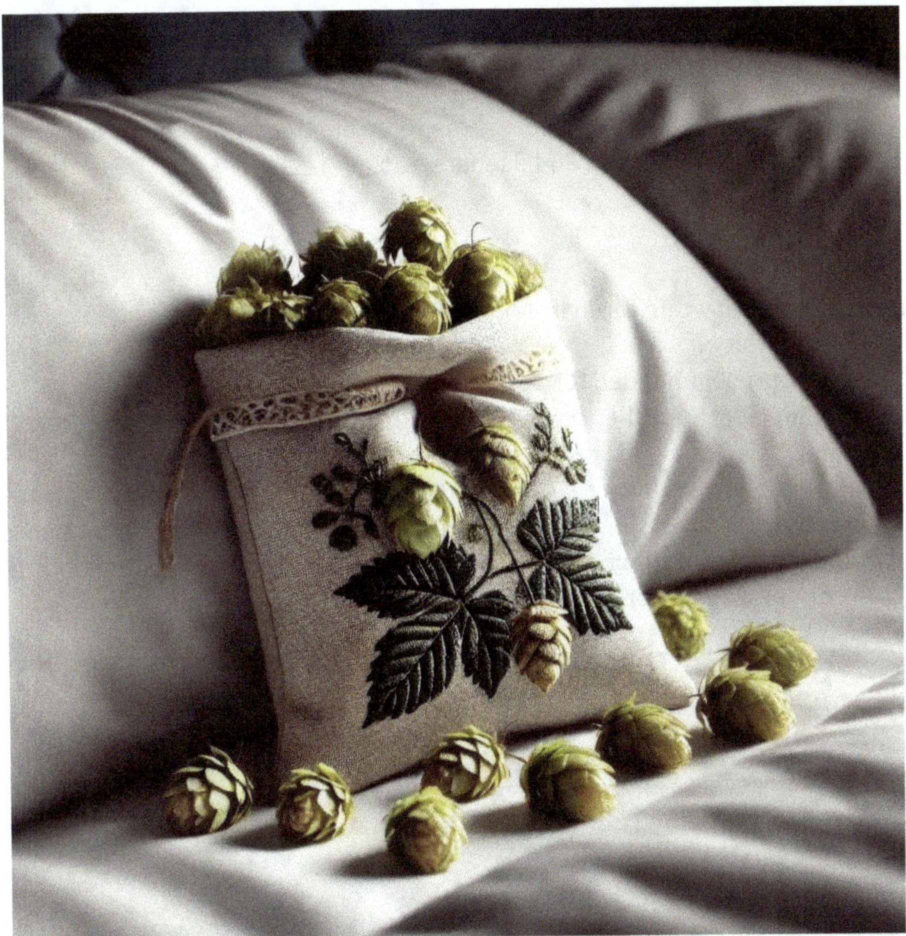

Ingredients:

- 1 cup dried hops flowers
- ½ cup dried lavender flowers (optional, for added scent)
- Small breathable fabric bags or squares of muslin cloth
- Ribbon or string to tie

1. In a bowl, combine the dried hops flowers and lavender if using.
2. Fill each fabric bag or place a portion of the mixture onto a muslin square.
3. If using muslin squares, gather the corners together and tie securely with ribbon or string to form a sachet.
4. Place the sachet inside your pillowcase or near your bed.

Usage:

Keep the sachet near your sleeping area to inhale the aroma throughout the night, promoting relaxation and deeper sleep.

Caution:

- Hops may cause skin irritation in sensitive individuals; discontinue use if irritation occurs.
- Not recommended for use during pregnancy.
- Replace the sachet contents every few weeks to maintain potency.

Note: These recipes aim to support relaxation and sleep through natural means. They are not a substitute for professional medical advice or treatment. If you experience chronic insomnia or anxiety, please consult a healthcare professional for appropriate care.

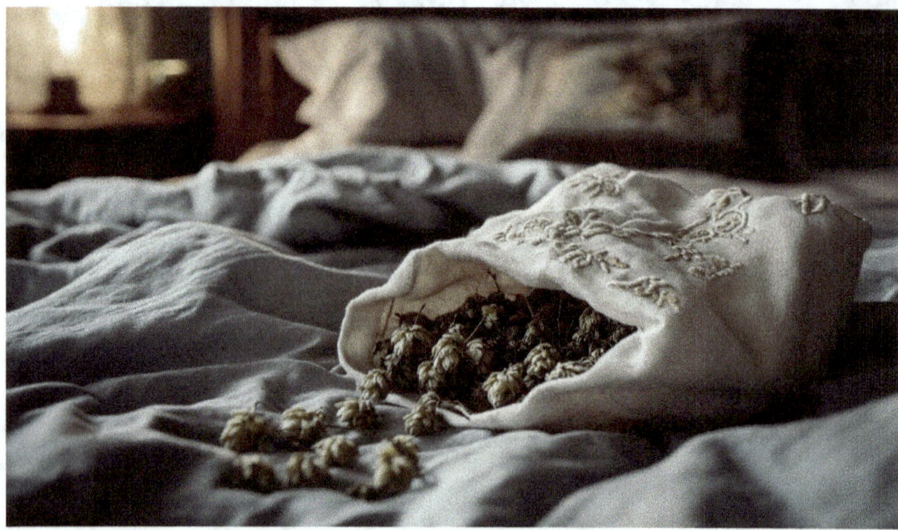

Recipe 16: Mullein Lung Support Tea

Mullein, a tall plant with soft, velvety leaves and bright yellow flowers, has been cherished for centuries for its soothing effects on the respiratory system. Traditionally used to address coughs and congestion, mullein is believed to help clear the lungs and ease breathing. This gentle herb offers a natural way to support respiratory comfort during times of need.

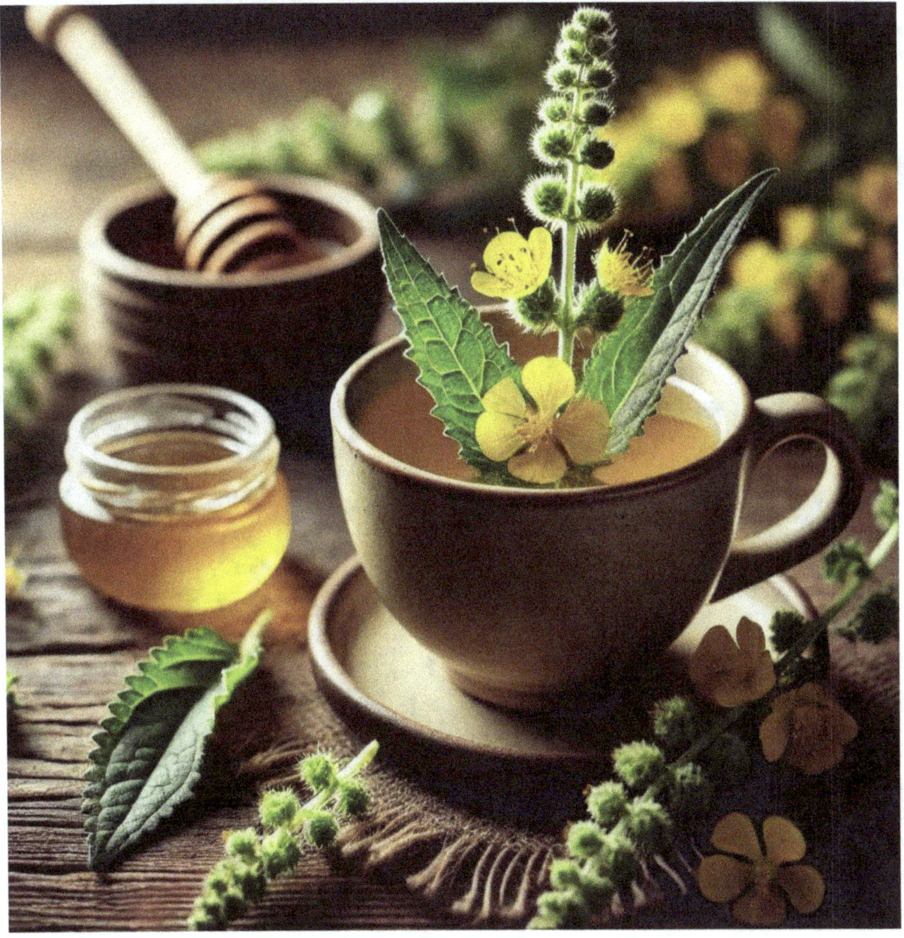

Ingredients:

- 2 teaspoons dried mullein leaves and flowers
- 1 cup boiling water
- Honey or lemon (optional, for taste)

1. Place the dried mullein in a tea infuser or teapot.
2. Pour boiling water over the herbs.
3. Cover and let steep for 10–15 minutes.
4. Strain the tea through a fine mesh strainer or cheesecloth to remove tiny hairs that may irritate the throat.
5. Add honey or lemon if desired.
6. Sip slowly while warm.

Drink up to three cups daily to support respiratory health and ease discomfort.

- Ensure thorough straining to remove fine plant hairs.
- Consult a healthcare professional if pregnant, nursing, or taking medications.
- Not recommended for long-term use without professional guidance.

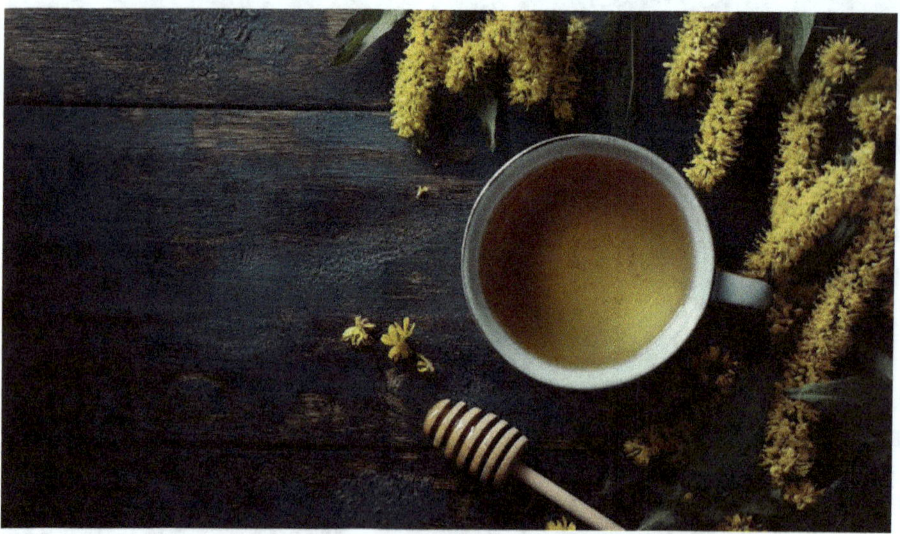

Recipe 17: Thyme Steam Inhalation for Congestion

Thyme, a fragrant herb commonly found in kitchens, holds powerful antimicrobial and expectorant properties. Inhaling thyme-infused steam can help loosen mucus, reduce nasal congestion, and soothe irritated airways. This simple remedy provides quick relief using ingredients readily available at home.

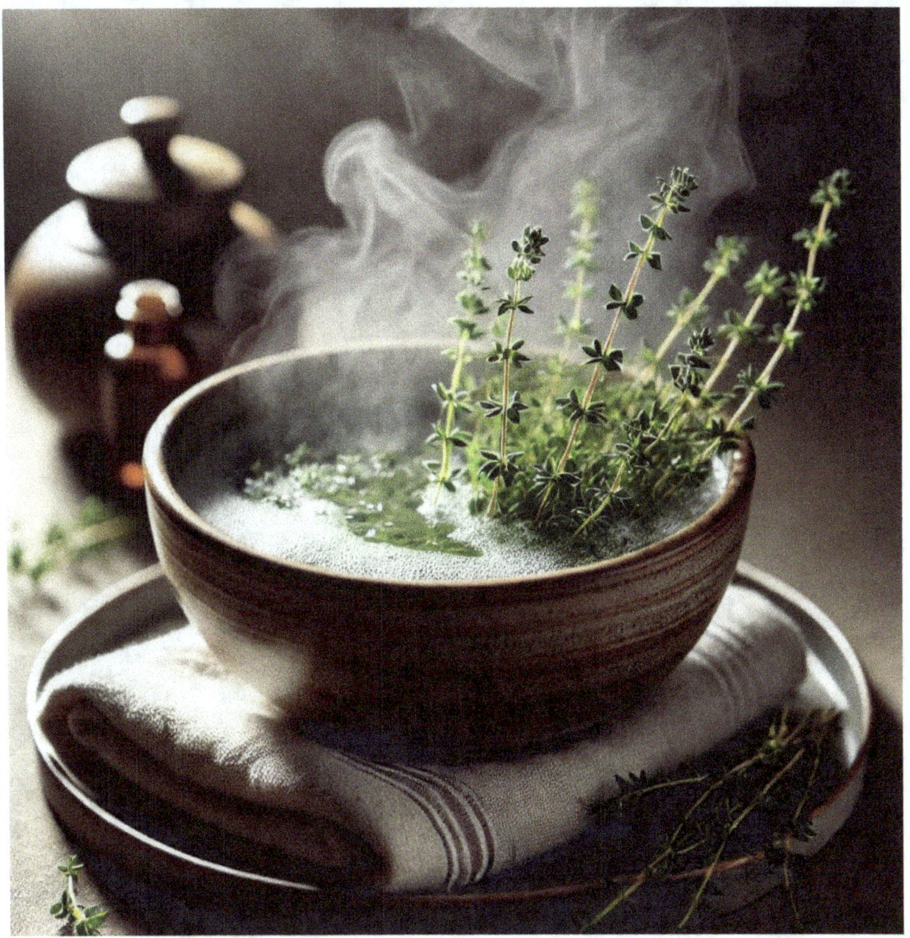

Ingredients:

- A handful of fresh thyme sprigs or 2 tablespoons dried thyme
- 4 cups boiling water
- Large bowl
- Towel

1. Place the thyme in a large, heat-resistant bowl.
2. Carefully pour boiling water over the herb.
3. Allow the mixture to cool slightly to a safe steaming temperature.
4. Lean over the bowl, keeping your face about 8–12 inches away.
5. Drape a towel over your head and the bowl to trap the steam.
6. Inhale deeply through your nose and mouth for 5–10 minutes.
7. Take breaks if necessary.

Usage:

Perform steam inhalation once or twice daily to alleviate congestion and support respiratory ease.

Caution:

- Use caution to avoid burns from hot steam.
- Keep eyes closed during inhalation.
- Not suitable for young children or individuals with asthma without professional advice.

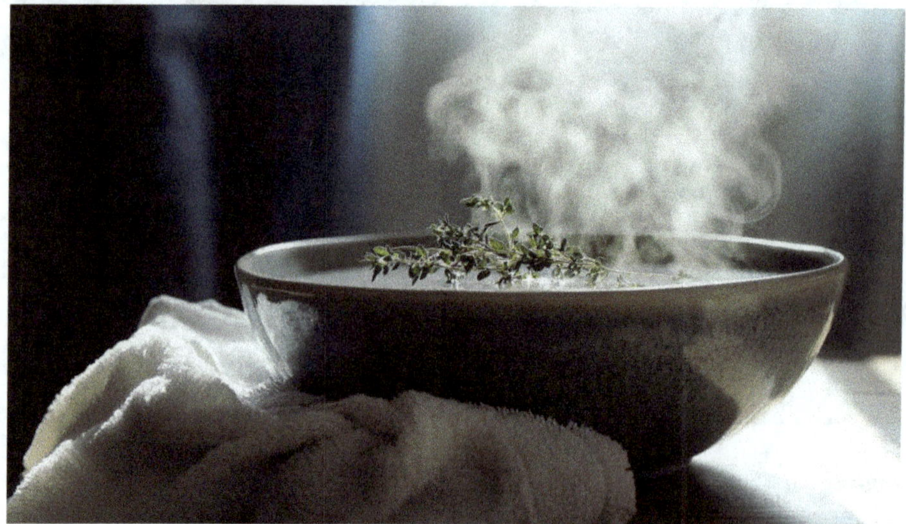

Recipe 18: Eucalyptus Chest Rub for Easy Breathing

Eucalyptus, native to Australia, is renowned for its invigorating scent and respiratory benefits. The essential oil derived from its leaves can help clear airways and ease breathing when applied topically. Crafting a homemade chest rub with eucalyptus offers a natural alternative to commercial vapor rubs.

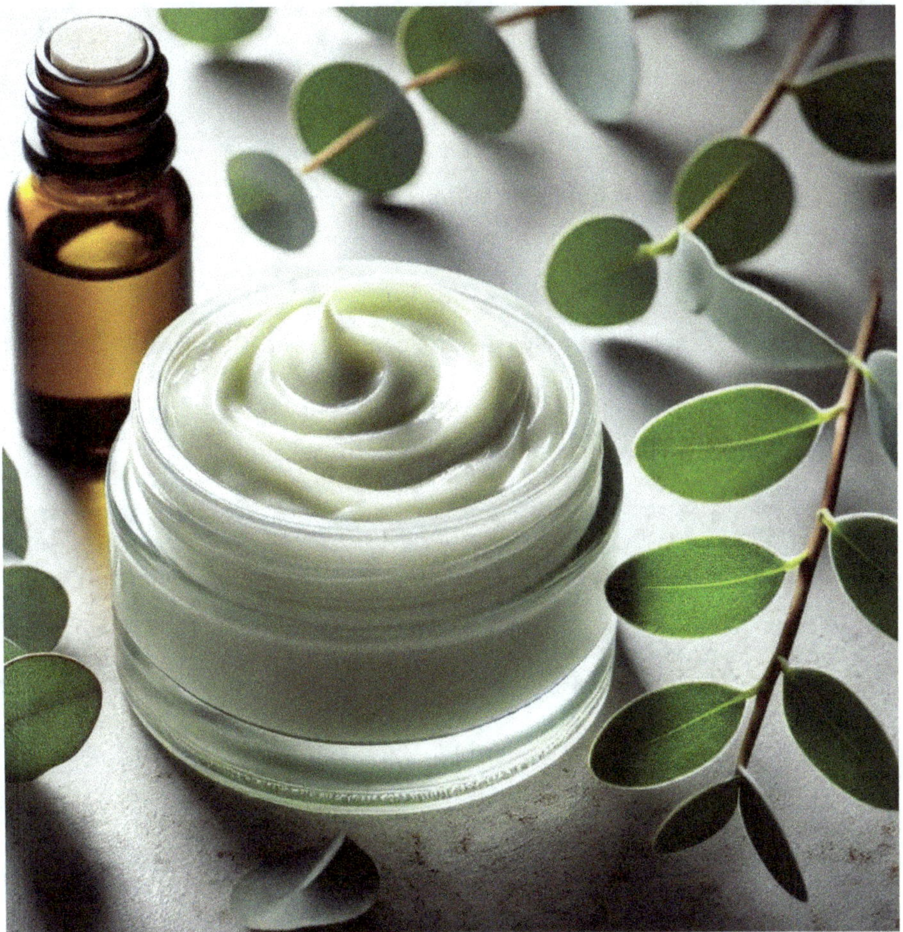

Ingredients:

- ½ cup coconut oil or shea butter
- 2 tablespoons beeswax pellets
- 20 drops eucalyptus essential oil
- 10 drops lavender or peppermint essential oil (optional)
- Small glass jar with lid

1. In a double boiler, melt the coconut oil (or shea butter) and beeswax over low heat.
2. Once melted, remove from heat and let cool slightly.
3. Stir in eucalyptus essential oil and optional essential oil if using.
4. Pour the mixture into the glass jar.
5. Allow it to cool and solidify completely before sealing.
6. Label the jar and store in a cool, dark place.

Usage:

Gently massage a small amount onto the chest and upper back to promote clear breathing, especially before bedtime.

Caution:

- For external use only; avoid contact with eyes and mucous membranes.
- Not suitable for children under two years of age.
- Test on a small skin area first to check for sensitivity.

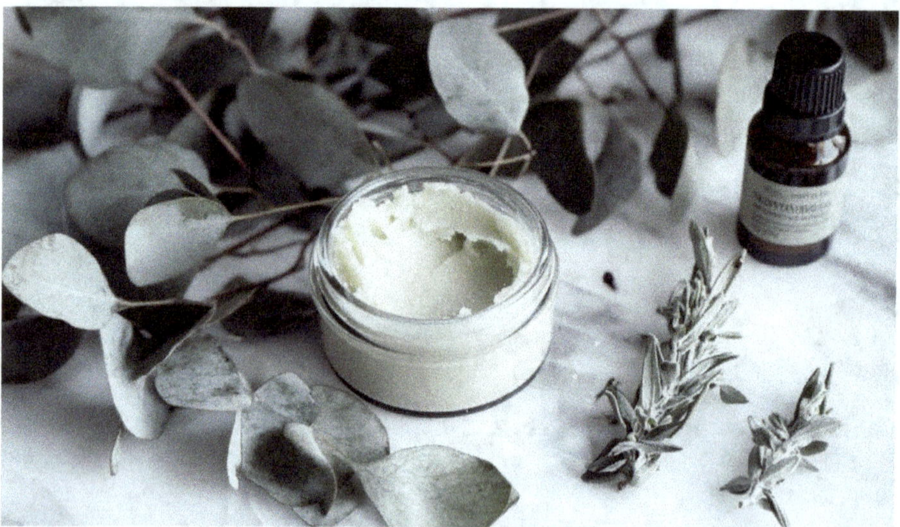

Recipe 19: Licorice Root Sore Throat Lozenges

Licorice root, with its naturally sweet flavor, has been a favored remedy for soothing sore throats and coughs. Its demulcent properties help coat mucous membranes, providing relief from irritation. Making your own lozenges allows you to harness the benefits of licorice root in a convenient form.

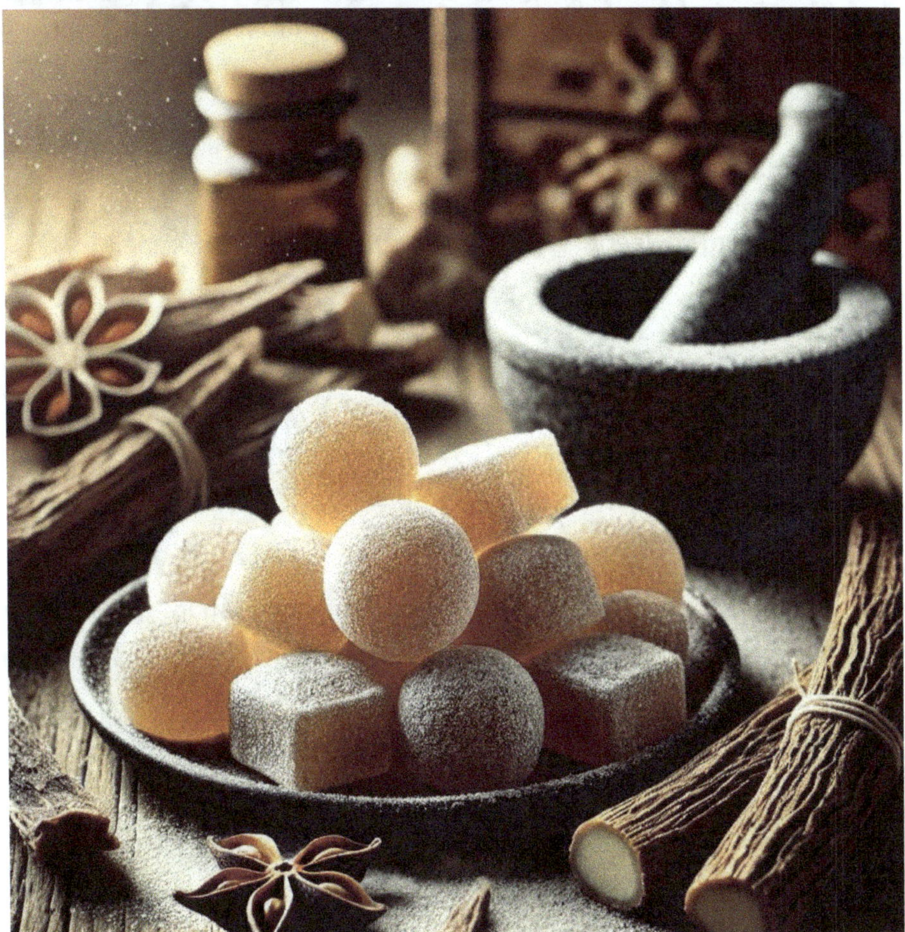

Ingredients:

- 1 cup strong licorice root tea (brew by simmering 2 tablespoons dried licorice root in 1½ cups water until reduced)
- 1 cup granulated sugar or ¾ cup honey
- 1 tablespoon lemon juice
- Powdered sugar or cornstarch for dusting
- Candy thermometer (if available)

Instructions:

1. Prepare licorice root tea and strain to obtain 1 cup of liquid.
2. In a saucepan, combine the licorice tea, sugar or honey, and lemon juice.
3. Stir over medium heat until sugar dissolves.
4. Bring to a boil and cook until the mixture reaches 300°F (hard crack stage) on a candy thermometer, or test by dropping a small amount into cold water—it should harden immediately.
5. Remove from heat and let bubbles subside.
6. Carefully spoon drops onto a parchment-lined baking sheet or pour into candy molds.
7. Allow lozenges to cool and harden completely.
8. Dust with powdered sugar or cornstarch to prevent sticking.
9. Store in an airtight container away from moisture.

Usage:

Dissolve one lozenge slowly in the mouth as needed to soothe throat discomfort.

Caution:

- Licorice root may interact with certain medications and is not recommended for people with high blood pressure, heart disease, or kidney issues.
- Avoid prolonged use without consulting a healthcare professional.
- Not suitable during pregnancy.

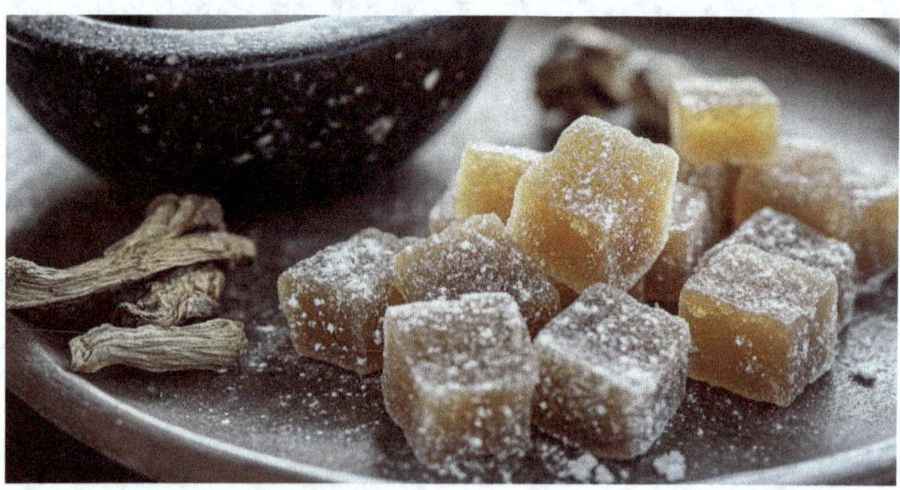

Recipe 20: Sage Gargle for Throat Soothing

Sage, an herb with a storied history, is celebrated for its antiseptic and anti-inflammatory properties. Used as a gargle, sage can help alleviate sore throat symptoms by reducing inflammation and combating bacteria. This simple yet effective remedy is a staple in natural throat care.

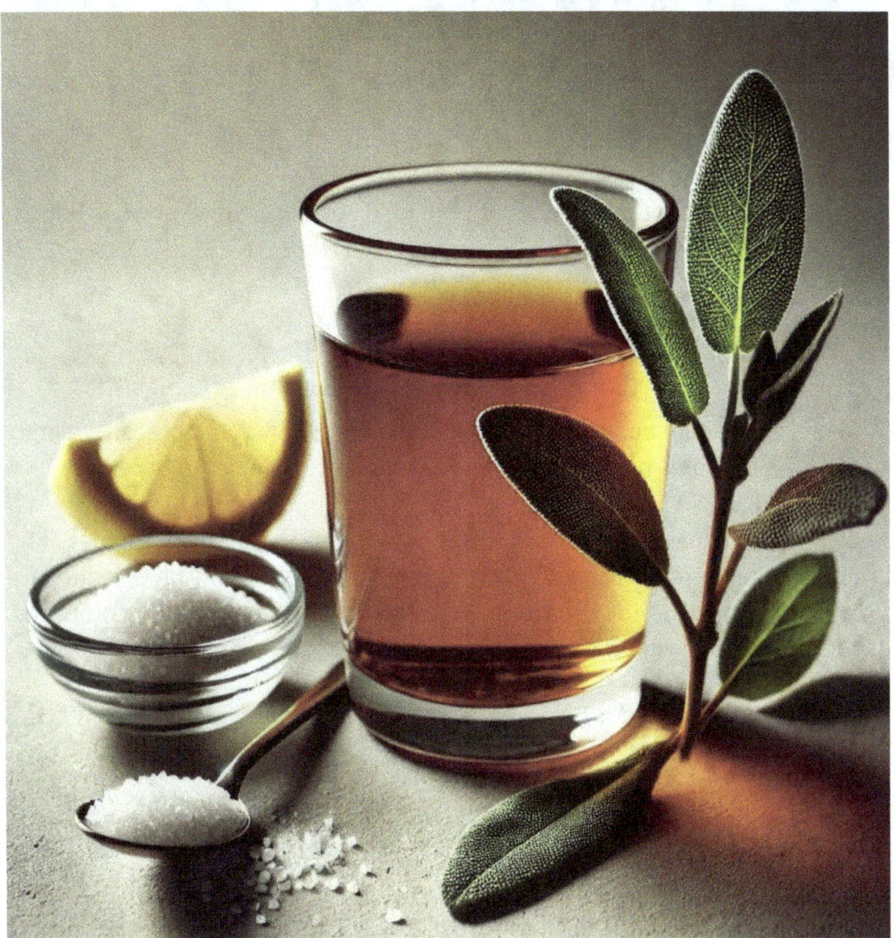

Ingredients:

- 2 teaspoons dried sage leaves or a handful of fresh leaves
- 1 cup boiling water
- ½ teaspoon sea salt
- Optional: 1 teaspoon apple cider vinegar or honey for added soothing effect

Instructions:

1. Place sage leaves in a heatproof cup or mug.
2. Pour boiling water over the leaves.
3. Cover and steep for 15 minutes.
4. Strain to remove the leaves.
5. Stir in sea salt until dissolved.
6. Add apple cider vinegar or honey if desired.
7. Allow the gargle to cool to a comfortable temperature.

Usage:

Gargle with a mouthful of the solution for 30 seconds, then spit out. Repeat several times daily as needed.

Caution:

- Do not swallow the gargle.
- Sage should be used cautiously during pregnancy and breastfeeding.
- If symptoms persist beyond a few days, seek medical advice.

Note: These recipes are intended to support general respiratory wellness and are not a substitute for professional medical care. Always consult a healthcare provider for persistent symptoms or before starting new health practices, especially if you have existing health conditions or are taking medications.

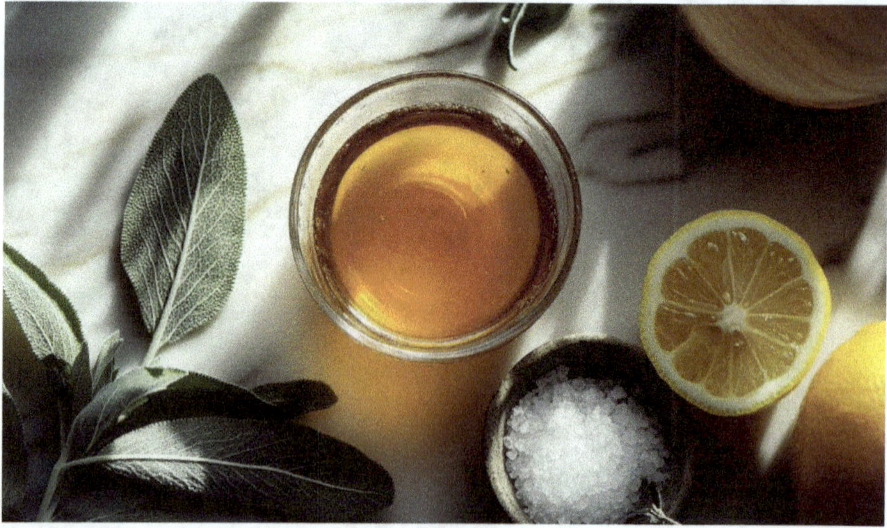

Recipe 21: Aloe Vera Skin Healing Gel

Aloe vera, often referred to as the "plant of immortality" by ancient Egyptians, is renowned for its soothing and healing properties. The clear gel found inside its thick leaves is packed with vitamins, minerals, and antioxidants that promote skin repair and hydration. Whether you're dealing with sunburn, minor cuts, or dry skin, homemade aloe vera gel is a versatile remedy for various skin ailments.

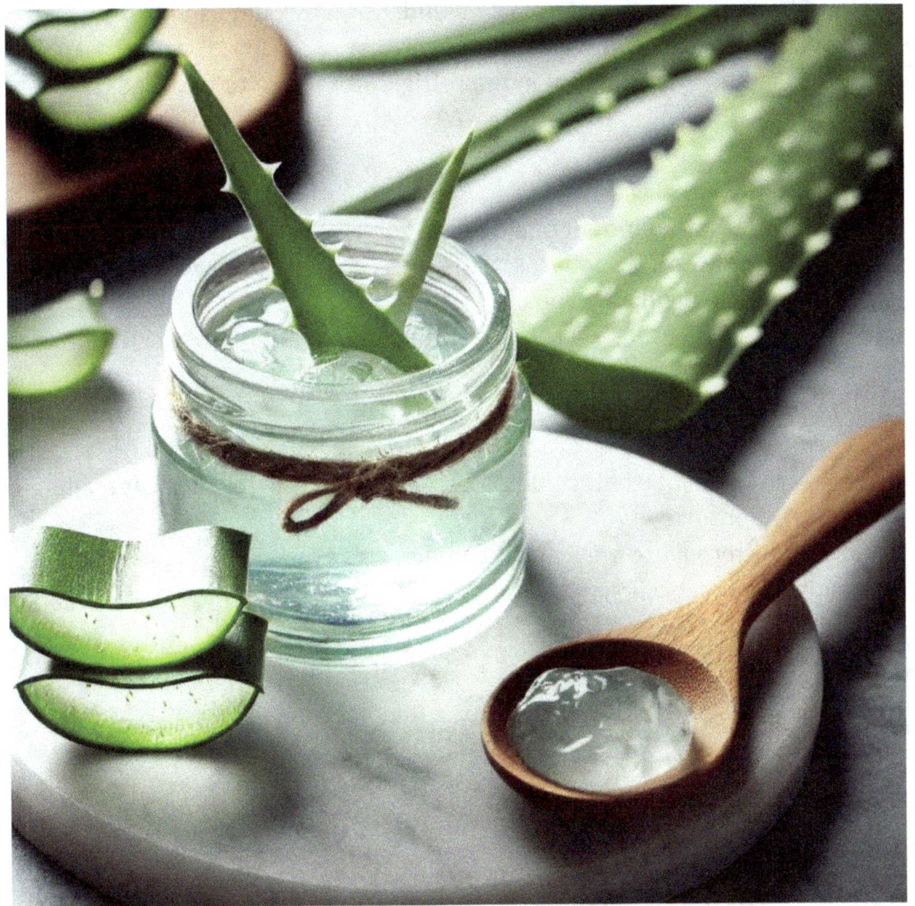

Ingredients:

- 2–3 large aloe vera leaves
- 500 mg of vitamin C powder or a few drops of vitamin E oil (optional, as a natural preservative)

- A clean glass jar with a lid

Instructions:

1. Wash the aloe vera leaves thoroughly to remove any dirt or debris.
2. Carefully cut off the serrated edges on both sides of each leaf.
3. Slice the top layer of the leaf lengthwise to expose the clear gel inside.
4. Using a spoon or spatula, gently scoop out the gel and place it into a clean bowl.
5. If using vitamin C powder or vitamin E oil, add it to the gel and mix well. This helps preserve the gel and adds extra antioxidant benefits.
6. Blend the gel mixture using a blender or whisk until smooth.
7. Transfer the gel into a sterilized glass jar.
8. Seal the jar and store it in the refrigerator for up to two weeks.

Usage:

- Apply a small amount of aloe vera gel directly to the skin as needed.
- Use it to soothe sunburns, moisturize dry skin, or promote healing of minor cuts and abrasions.
- Can also be used as a calming facial mask or aftershave balm.

Caution:

- Perform a patch test before widespread use to check for allergic reactions.
- For external use only; avoid contact with eyes.
- If irritation occurs, discontinue use.

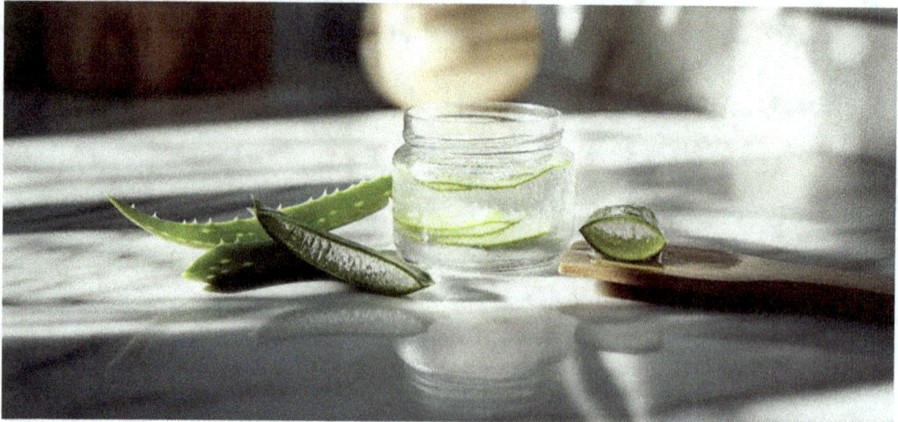

Recipe 22: Calendula Antiseptic Salve

Calendula, also known as marigold, has been treasured for its healing properties since the Middle Ages. The vibrant orange and yellow petals contain flavonoids and triterpenoids, compounds that provide anti-inflammatory and antiseptic effects. A homemade calendula salve is an excellent natural remedy for cuts, scrapes, insect bites, and other minor skin irritations.

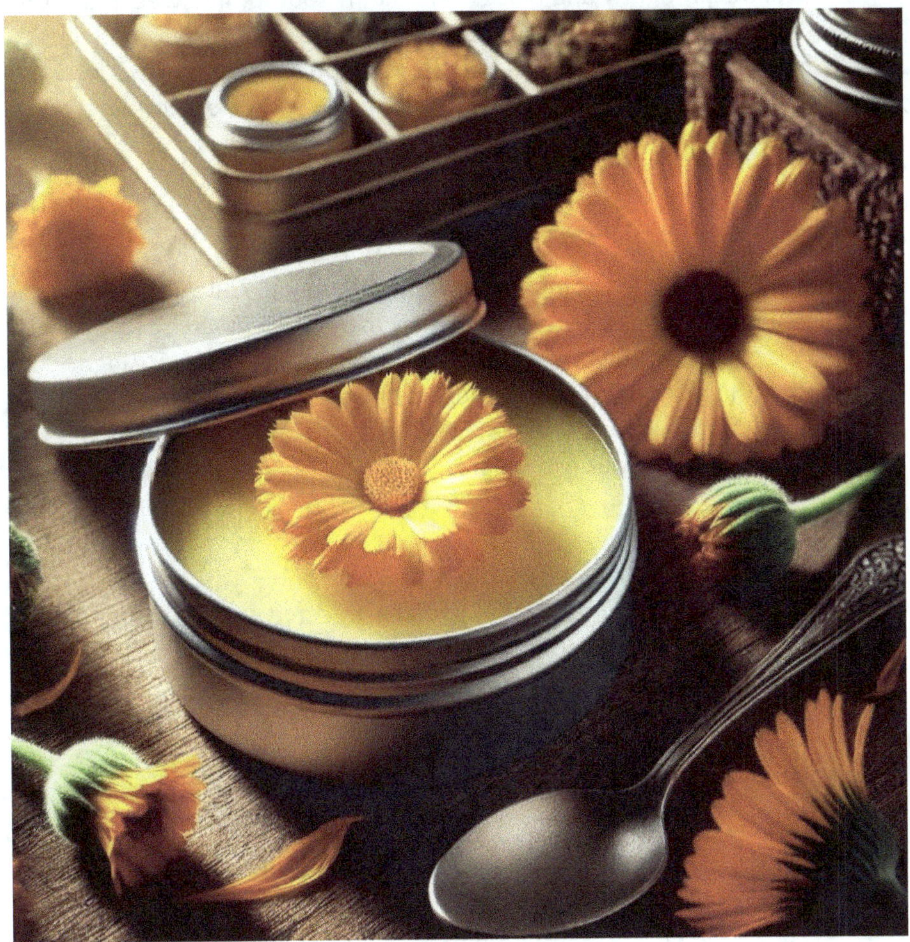

Ingredients:

- 1 cup dried calendula petals
- 1 cup olive oil or sweet almond oil
- ¼ cup beeswax pellets
- Optional: 10 drops lavender essential oil for added soothing properties
- Sterilized glass jars or tins for storage

Infuse the Oil:

1. Place the dried calendula petals in a clean, dry glass jar.
2. Pour the olive oil over the petals, ensuring they are completely submerged.
3. Seal the jar tightly and place it in a sunny spot for 4–6 weeks, shaking it gently every few days. Alternatively, for a quicker method, gently heat the oil and petals in a double boiler on low heat for 2–3 hours.
4. After infusion, strain the oil through a cheesecloth or fine mesh strainer into a clean bowl, squeezing out as much oil as possible.

Make the Salve:

5. In a double boiler, combine the infused calendula oil and beeswax.
6. Heat gently until the beeswax is fully melted, stirring occasionally.
7. Remove from heat and stir in the lavender essential oil if using.
8. Pour the mixture into sterilized jars or tins.
9. Allow the salve to cool and solidify completely before sealing.
10. Label and date your containers.

Usage:

- Apply a small amount of salve to clean, affected areas 2–3 times daily.
- Use for minor cuts, scrapes, dry skin patches, and insect bites.
- Can also serve as a nourishing hand or foot balm.

Caution:

- For external use only.
- Perform a patch test to ensure no allergic reactions.
- Avoid use if allergic to plants in the Asteraceae/Compositae family (e.g., ragweed, chrysanthemums).

Recipe 23: Rosemary Hair Strengthening Rinse

Rosemary, a fragrant herb native to the Mediterranean, has been associated with memory enhancement and hair health for centuries. Its stimulating properties can help improve scalp circulation, potentially promoting hair growth and strengthening follicles. A rosemary rinse adds shine and vitality to hair, making it a simple yet effective addition to your hair care routine.

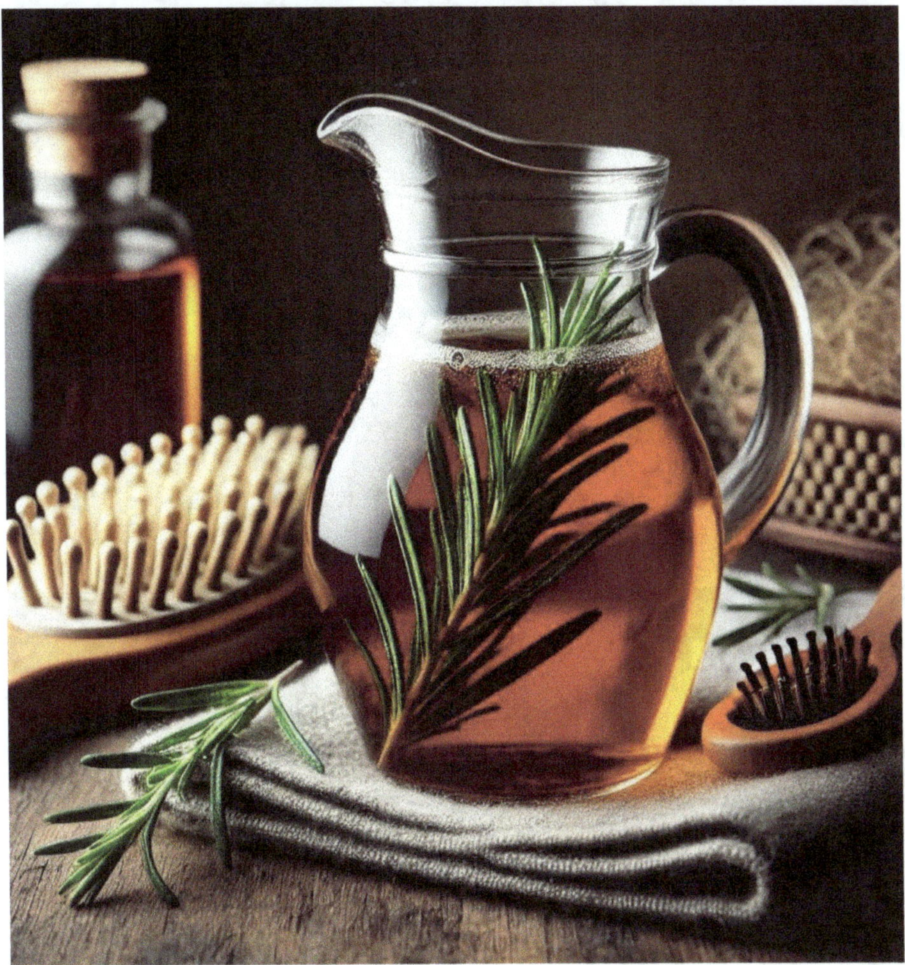

Ingredients:

- 2 cups water
- 3–4 sprigs of fresh rosemary or 2 tablespoons dried rosemary
- Optional: 1 tablespoon apple cider vinegar for extra shine

Instructions:

1. Bring the water to a boil in a saucepan.
2. Add the rosemary to the boiling water.
3. Reduce heat and simmer for 10–15 minutes.
4. Remove from heat, cover, and let steep until the mixture cools to a comfortable temperature.
5. Strain the liquid into a pitcher or large bowl.
6. Stir in apple cider vinegar if desired.

Usage:

- After shampooing and rinsing your hair, slowly pour the rosemary rinse over your scalp and hair.
- Massage gently to ensure even distribution.
- Do not rinse out; simply towel dry and style as usual.
- Use once or twice a week for best results.

Caution:

- Avoid contact with eyes.
- If you have very light-colored hair, test on a small section first, as rosemary may darken hair over time.

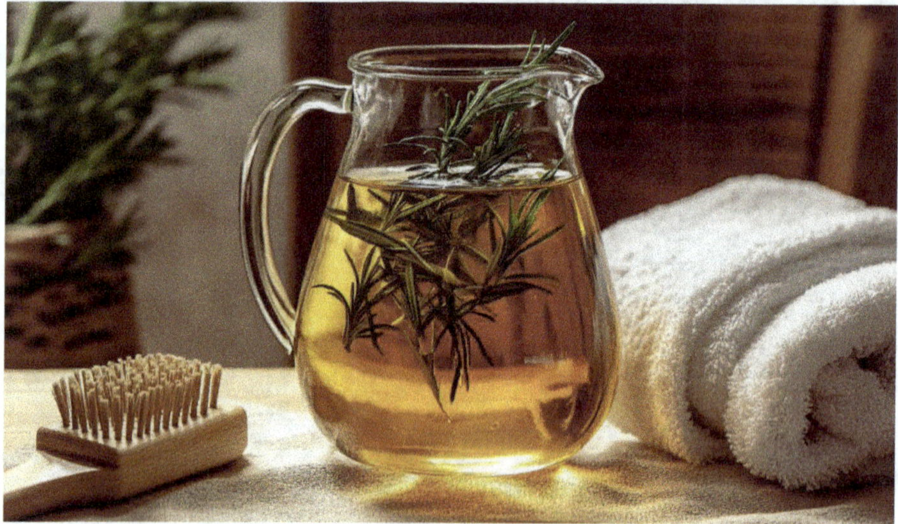

Recipe 24: Nettle Leaf Hair Growth Tonic

Stinging nettle, despite its prickly reputation, is a powerhouse of nutrients beneficial for hair health. Rich in vitamins A, C, K, and minerals like silica and iron, nettle can help strengthen hair, reduce hair loss, and encourage new growth. Creating a nettle hair tonic is an excellent way to harness these benefits naturally.

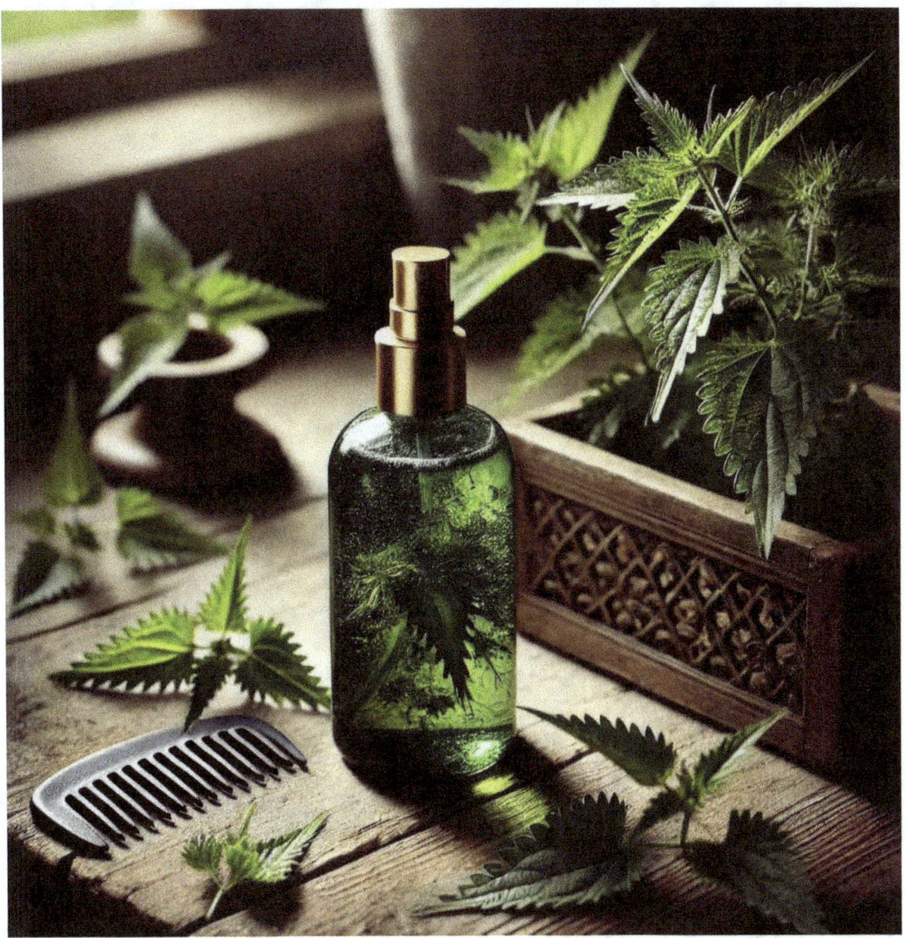

Ingredients:

- 2 cups water
- 1 cup fresh nettle leaves or 2 tablespoons dried nettle leaves
- Optional: 10 drops rosemary essential oil for added benefits
- Spray bottle for application

Instructions:

1. Wear gloves to handle fresh nettle leaves to avoid stings.
2. In a saucepan, bring water to a boil.
3. Add nettle leaves to the boiling water.
4. Reduce heat and simmer for 15–20 minutes.
5. Remove from heat, cover, and let steep until completely cool.
6. Strain the liquid into a bowl.
7. Add rosemary essential oil if using and stir well.
8. Transfer the tonic into a clean spray bottle.

Usage:

- Spray the tonic onto your scalp and hair roots, massaging gently.
- Leave it in; no need to rinse.
- Use daily or at least three times a week for optimal results.

Caution:

- Perform a patch test to ensure no allergic reactions.
- If irritation occurs, discontinue use.
- Store tonic in the refrigerator and use within one week.

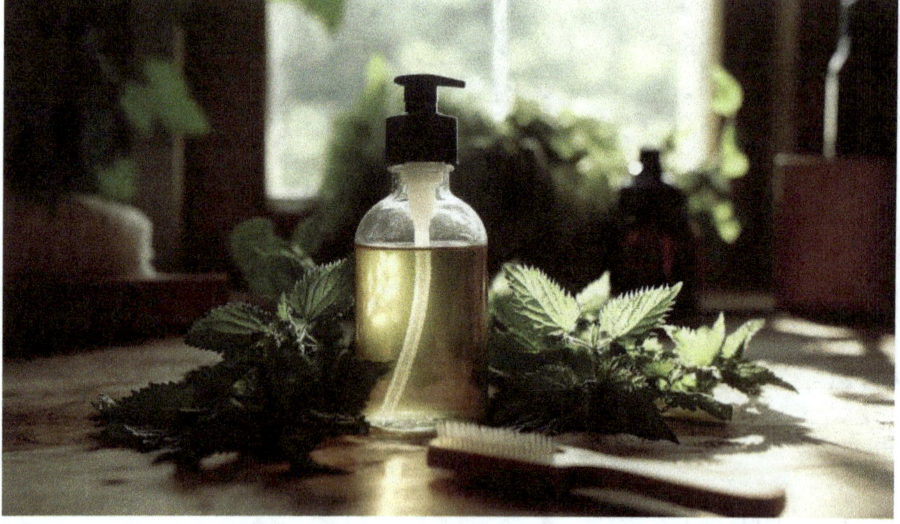

Recipe 25: Tea Tree Oil Acne Treatment

Tea tree oil, derived from the leaves of the Melaleuca alternifolia plant native to Australia, is famed for its potent antibacterial and anti-inflammatory properties. It has been used traditionally to treat various skin conditions, including acne. A diluted tea tree oil solution can help reduce acne-causing bacteria and soothe inflamed skin.

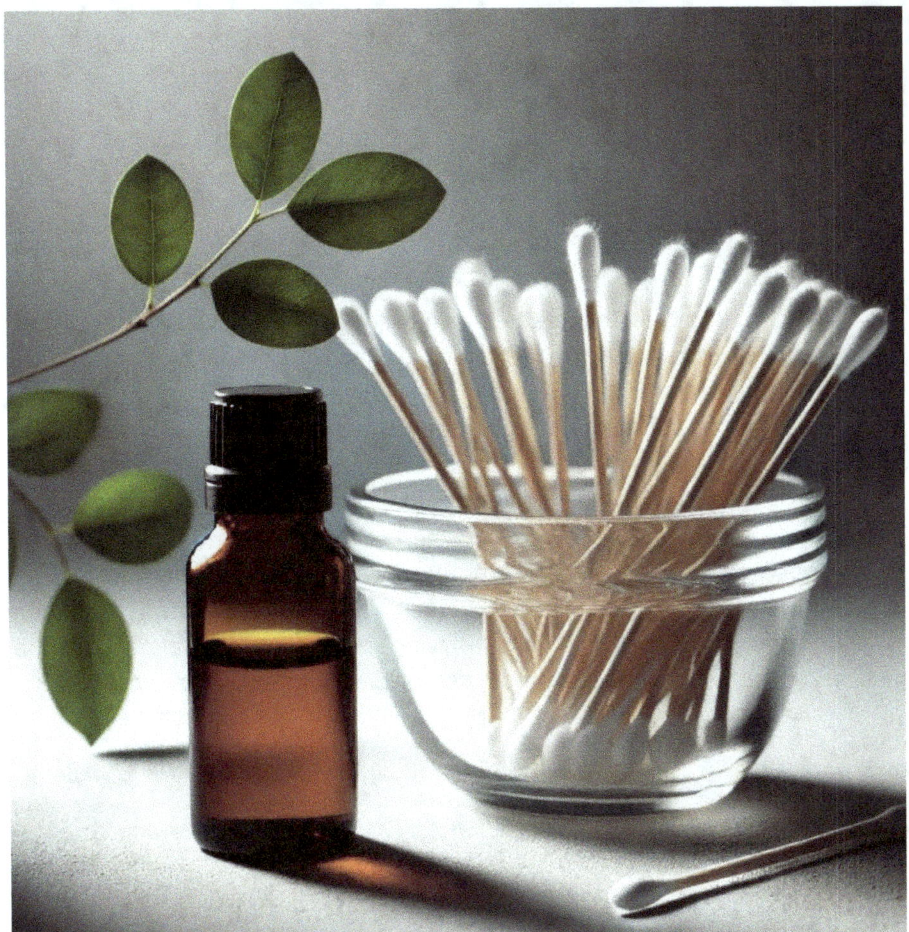

Ingredients:

- 1 teaspoon tea tree essential oil
- 9 teaspoons carrier oil (e.g., jojoba oil, grapeseed oil) or distilled water for dilution
- Clean cotton swabs or pads
- Small glass bottle for storage

Instructions:

1. In the glass bottle, combine tea tree oil with the carrier oil or distilled water to create a 10% dilution.
2. Shake well to mix thoroughly.
3. Label the bottle with the contents and date.

Usage:

- Cleanse your face thoroughly.
- Dip a cotton swab or pad into the diluted tea tree oil solution.
- Apply directly to acne spots or blemishes once or twice daily.
- Allow it to dry before applying moisturizer or makeup.

Caution:

- Do not use undiluted tea tree oil directly on the skin to avoid irritation.
- For external use only; avoid contact with eyes and mucous membranes.
- Not recommended for use during pregnancy or on young children without professional advice.
- Discontinue use if skin irritation or allergic reaction occurs.

Note: These natural remedies aim to support skin and hair health through gentle, plant-based ingredients. However, individual reactions can vary. Always perform a patch test when trying a new product and consult a healthcare professional or dermatologist for persistent or severe conditions.

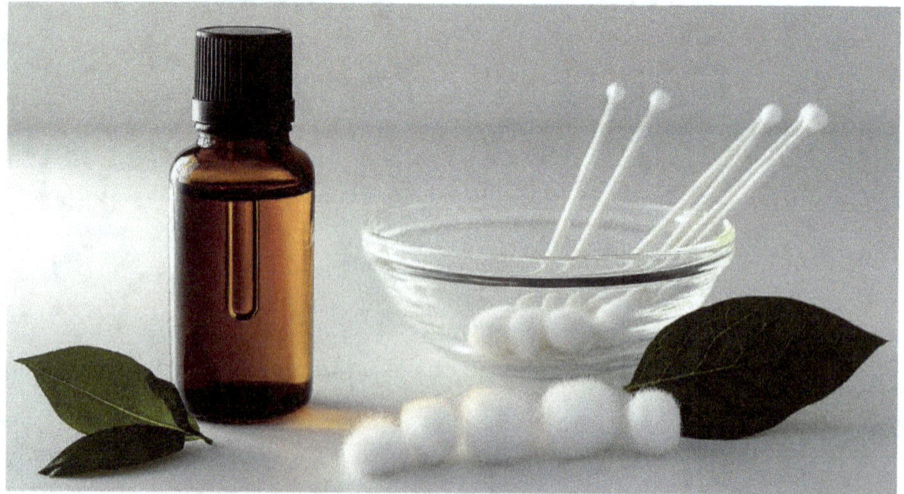

Recipe 26: Red Raspberry Leaf Uterine Tonic Tea

For centuries, red raspberry leaf has been cherished by women for its reputed ability to support reproductive health. Native to Europe and parts of Asia, this herb is rich in vitamins and minerals, particularly iron, which is essential for women's well-being. Traditionally used to tone the uterine muscles, red raspberry leaf tea is a gentle way to nourish the female body, especially during pregnancy and menstrual cycles.

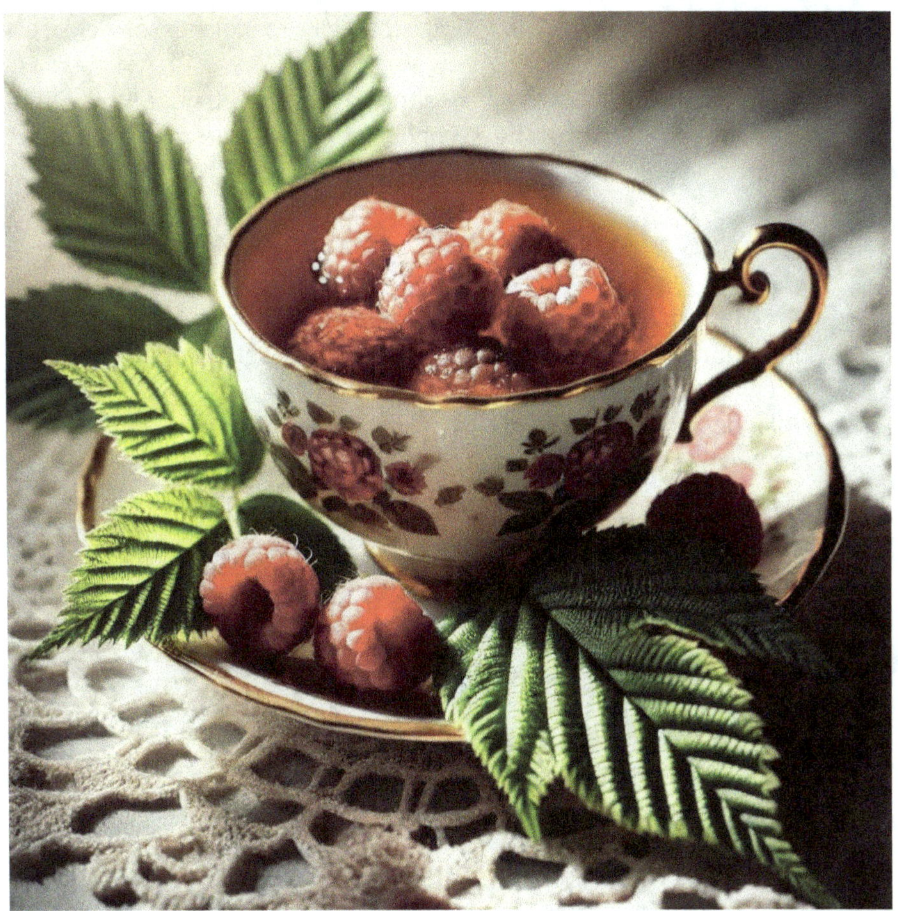

Ingredients:

- 1 tablespoon dried red raspberry leaves
- 1 cup boiling water
- Honey or lemon to taste (optional)

1. Place the dried red raspberry leaves in a teapot or infuser.
2. Pour boiling water over the leaves.
3. Cover and let steep for 10–15 minutes.
4. Strain the tea into a cup.
5. Add honey or lemon if desired.
6. Sip slowly and enjoy the soothing effects.

- **Menstrual Support:** Drink 1–3 cups daily to help ease menstrual discomfort.
- **Pregnancy:** Consult with a healthcare provider before use. Often recommended during the second and third trimesters to support uterine health.

- **Pregnancy:** While red raspberry leaf is generally considered safe, it's important to consult a healthcare professional before use during pregnancy, especially in the first trimester.
- **Allergies:** Avoid if allergic to plants in the Rosaceae family (e.g., strawberries, apples).

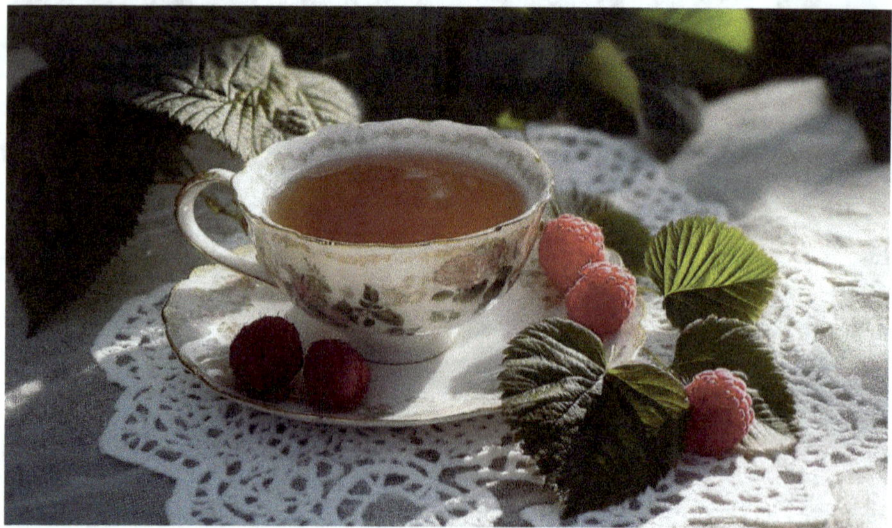

Recipe 27: Chasteberry Hormone Balancing Tincture

Chasteberry, also known as Vitex agnus-castus, has a long history of use in supporting hormonal balance in women. Native to the Mediterranean region, this small fruit is believed to influence the pituitary gland, helping to regulate menstrual cycles and alleviate symptoms of PMS. A tincture made from chasteberry provides a concentrated form that's easy to incorporate into daily routines.

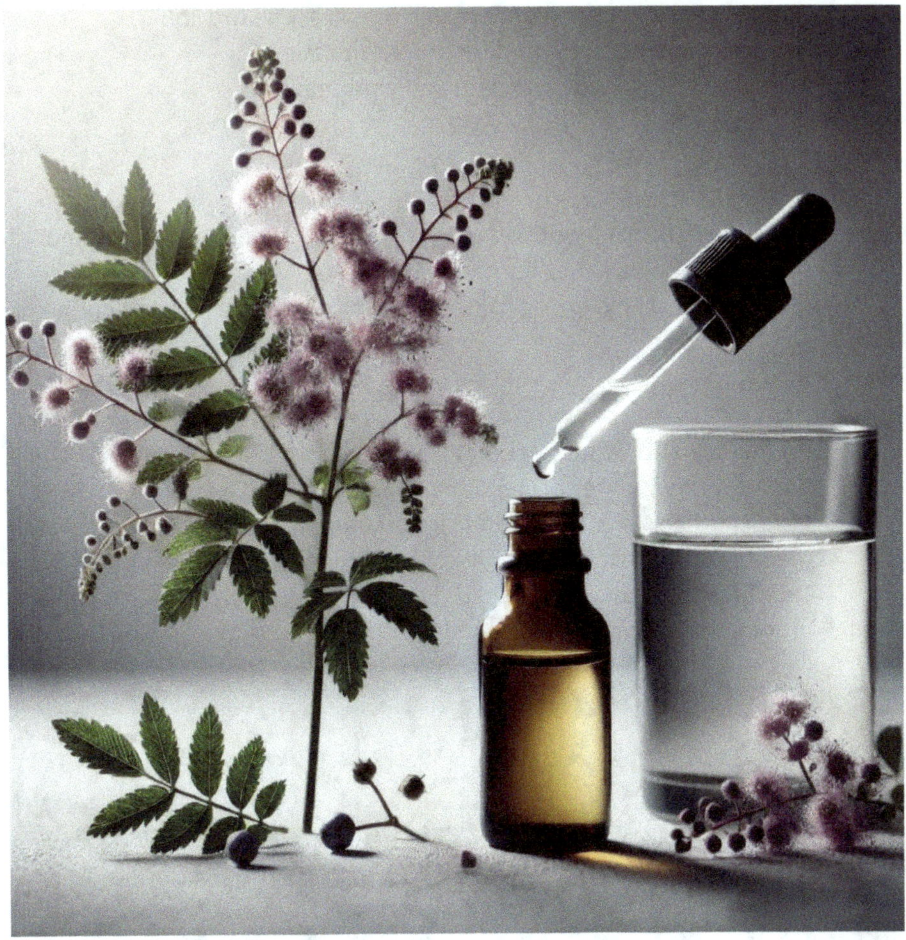

Ingredients:

- 1 cup dried chasteberries
- 2 cups vodka or brandy (80 proof)
- Clean glass jar with tight-fitting lid
- Dark glass dropper bottles for storage

1. Place the dried chasteberries in the glass jar.
2. Pour the alcohol over the berries, ensuring they are fully submerged with an extra inch of liquid above.
3. Seal the jar tightly and label it with the date and contents.
4. Store in a cool, dark place for 6–8 weeks, shaking gently every few days.
5. After steeping, strain the liquid through cheesecloth or a fine mesh strainer into a clean bowl, pressing to extract all the liquid.
6. Transfer the tincture into dark dropper bottles.
7. Label the bottles with the date and contents.

Usage:

- Take 30–40 drops (approximately 1–2 droppers full) in a small amount of water once daily in the morning.
- Consistency is key; it may take several months to notice effects.

Caution:

- **Pregnancy and Breastfeeding:** Do not use during pregnancy or while nursing unless under professional guidance.
- **Medications:** Consult a healthcare provider if taking hormone-related medications, birth control pills, or undergoing fertility treatments.
- **Side Effects:** May include mild digestive discomfort or skin reactions in some individuals.

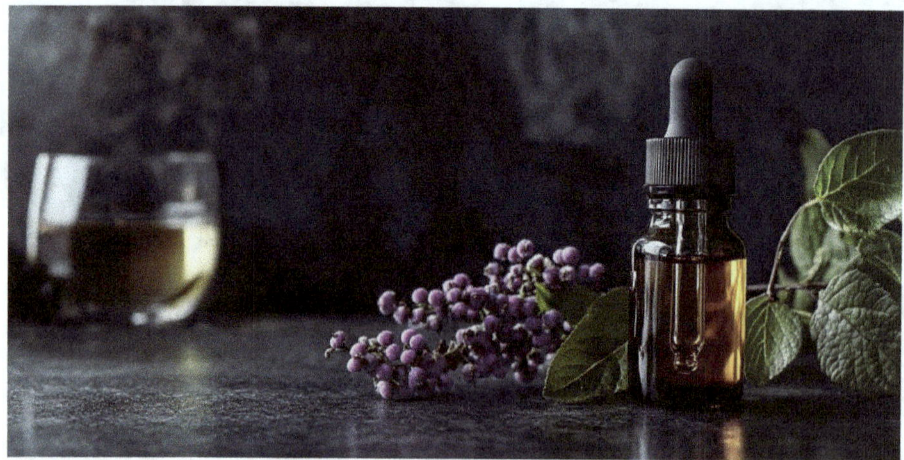

Recipe 28: Dong Quai Menstrual Comfort Decoction

Dong Quai, often referred to as the "female ginseng," is a traditional Chinese herb used for over a thousand years to support women's health. Known for its potential to help balance hormones and improve blood circulation, Dong Quai may alleviate menstrual cramps and discomfort. Crafting a decoction unlocks the herb's beneficial compounds, providing a warming and restorative tonic.

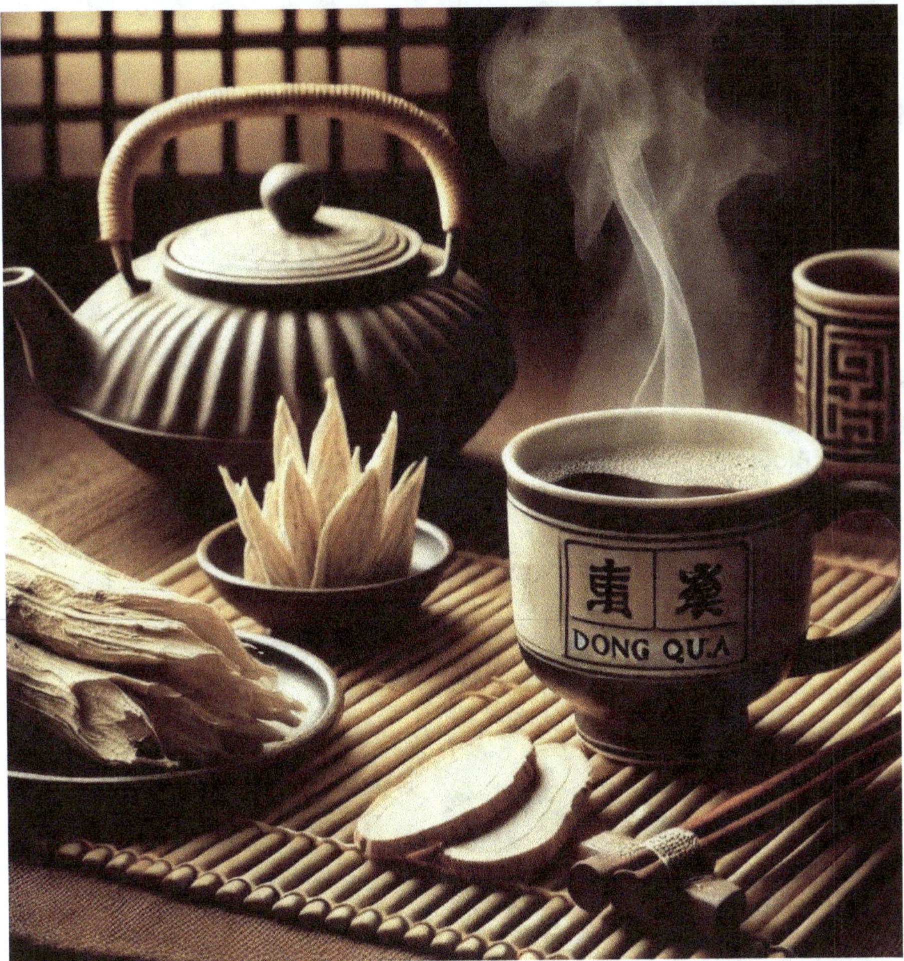

Ingredients:

- 1 tablespoon sliced dried Dong Quai root
- 2 cups water
- Optional: A slice of fresh ginger for added warmth

Instructions:

1. In a saucepan, combine the Dong Quai root (and ginger if using) with water.
2. Bring to a boil over medium heat.
3. Reduce heat and simmer gently for 20–30 minutes.
4. Remove from heat and strain the liquid into a cup.
5. Discard the herbs.
6. Allow to cool slightly before drinking.

Usage:

- Drink one cup daily during the week leading up to menstruation to help reduce discomfort.
- Can be consumed warm or at room temperature.

Caution:

- **Pregnancy:** Do not use during pregnancy, as Dong Quai may stimulate uterine contractions.
- **Blood Thinners:** Avoid if taking anticoagulant medications or have bleeding disorders.
- **Sun Sensitivity:** May increase sensitivity to sunlight; wear sunscreen if spending extended time outdoors.

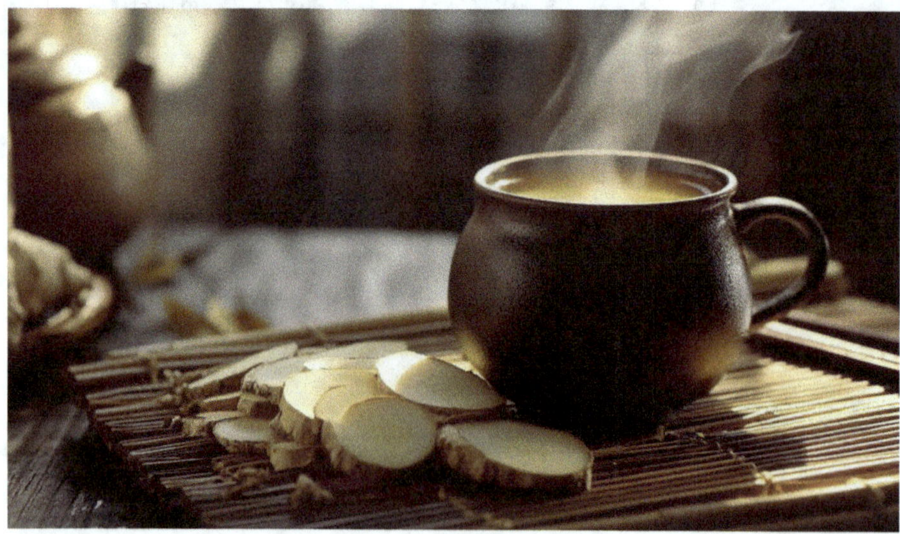

Recipe 29: Evening Primrose Oil Capsules for PMS

Evening primrose oil, extracted from the seeds of the evening primrose plant, is rich in gamma-linolenic acid (GLA), an essential fatty acid that may help balance hormones. Traditionally used to alleviate symptoms of premenstrual syndrome (PMS) such as breast tenderness, mood swings, and bloating, evening primrose oil offers a natural approach to monthly comfort.

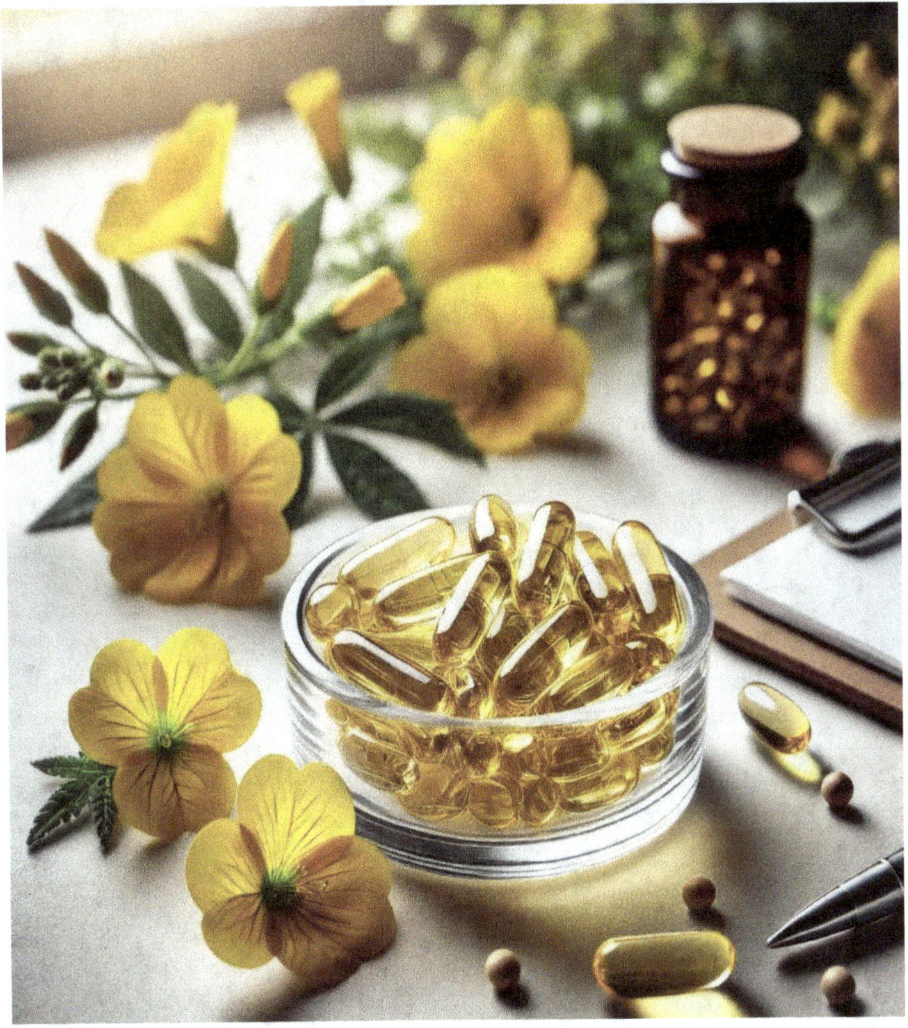

Ingredients:

- Evening primrose oil capsules (500 mg or as directed on the product)

Instructions:

1. Purchase high-quality evening primrose oil capsules from a reputable source.
2. Follow the dosage instructions on the packaging or as advised by a healthcare professional.

Usage:

- Common dosage is 1–3 capsules daily, starting one to two weeks before menstruation.
- Swallow capsules with water, preferably with meals.

Caution:

- **Medical Conditions:** Consult a healthcare provider if you have epilepsy, schizophrenia, or are taking medications that lower the seizure threshold.
- **Surgery:** Discontinue use two weeks before scheduled surgery due to potential blood-thinning effects.
- **Pregnancy and Breastfeeding:** Consult a healthcare professional before use.

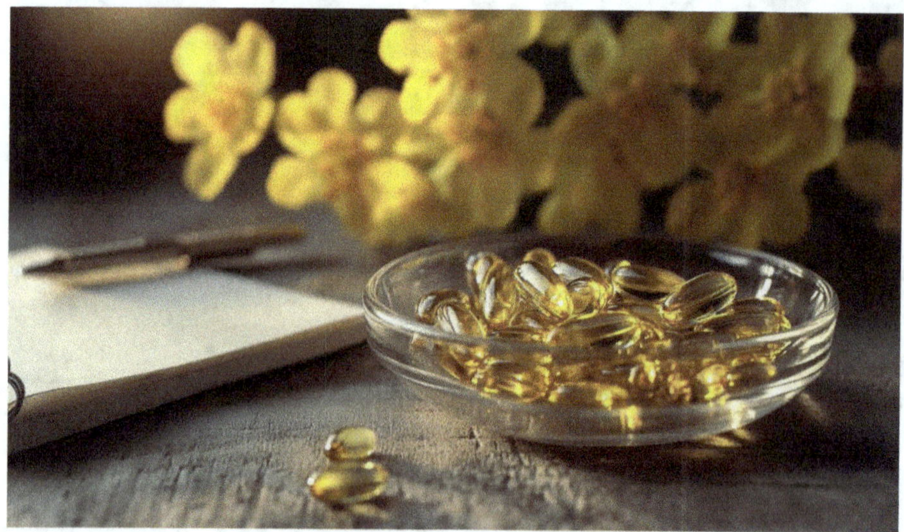

Recipe 30: Motherwort Emotional Support Tea

Motherwort, bearing the Latin name *Leonurus cardiaca*, meaning "lion's heart," has been used since ancient times to support women's emotional well-being, particularly related to the heart and stress. This herb is believed to help ease anxiety, calm nervous tension, and provide comfort during hormonal transitions such as menopause.

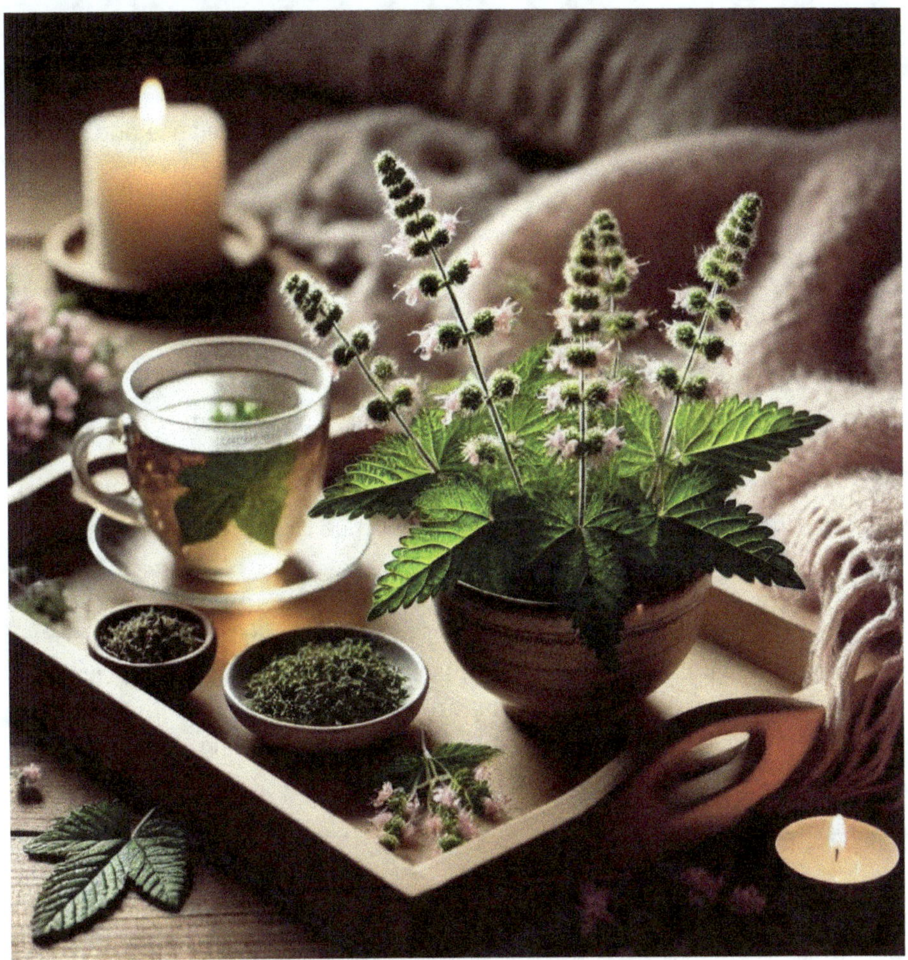

Ingredients:

- 1 teaspoon dried motherwort herb
- 1 cup boiling water
- Honey or sweetener of choice (optional)

1. Place the dried motherwort in a teapot or infuser.
2. Pour boiling water over the herb.
3. Cover and let steep for 10 minutes.
4. Strain the tea into a cup.
5. Add honey if desired to offset the herb's natural bitterness.
6. Enjoy slowly, embracing a moment of relaxation.

Usage:

- Drink up to two cups daily to support emotional balance and reduce feelings of anxiety.
- Ideal during times of stress or hormonal shifts.

Caution:

- **Pregnancy:** Do not use during pregnancy due to potential uterine stimulating effects.
- **Medications:** May interact with heart medications or sedatives; consult a healthcare provider.
- **Taste Profile:** Motherwort is naturally bitter; consider blending with other herbs like peppermint or chamomile to improve flavor.

Note: The herbal remedies in this chapter are intended to support general women's health and are not substitutes for professional medical advice or treatment. Individual responses to herbs can vary. It's important to consult a qualified healthcare professional before starting any new supplement or herbal regimen, especially during pregnancy, breastfeeding, or if you have underlying health conditions.

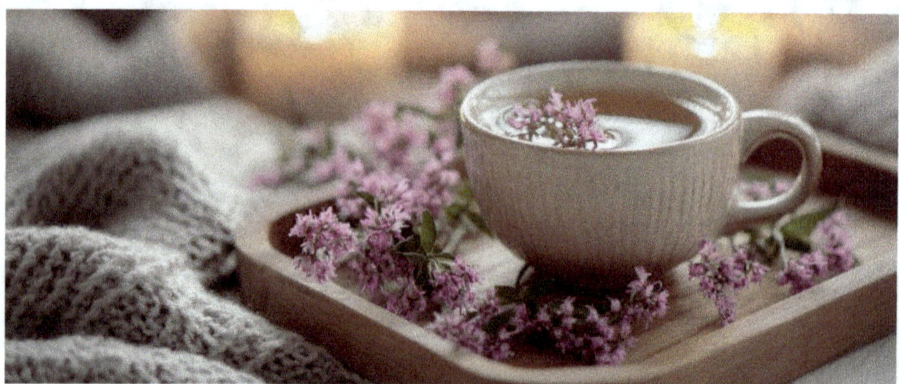

Recipe 31: Saw Palmetto Prostate Health Tea

Saw palmetto, a small palm native to the southeastern United States, has been used for centuries by Native American tribes to support men's health. Modern research highlights its potential in promoting prostate health and alleviating symptoms of benign prostatic hyperplasia (BPH). A soothing tea made from saw palmetto berries is a natural way to support urinary and reproductive well-being.

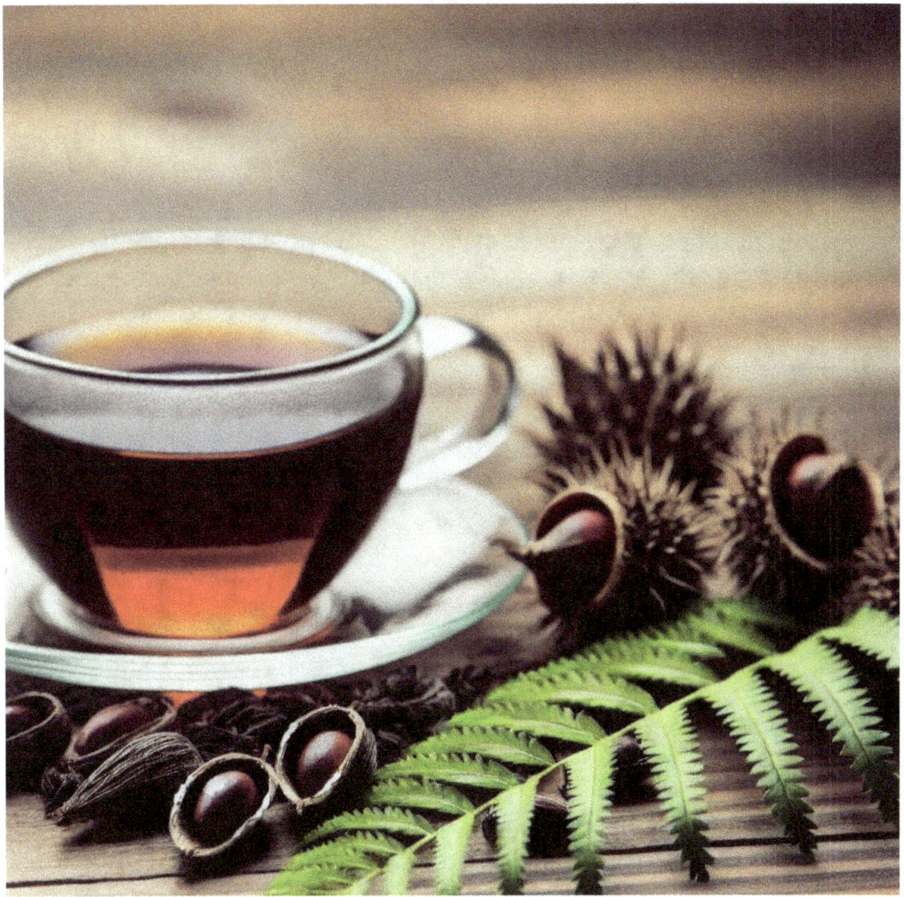

Ingredients:

- 1 tablespoon dried saw palmetto berries
- 1 cup boiling water
- Honey or lemon for taste (optional)

1. Place the dried saw palmetto berries in a teapot or infuser.
2. Pour boiling water over the berries.
3. Cover and let steep for 10–15 minutes.
4. Strain the tea into a cup.
5. Add honey or lemon if desired for flavor.
6. Sip slowly, enjoying the earthy richness of the tea.

Usage:

- Drink one cup daily to support prostate and urinary health.
- Consult with a healthcare provider for long-term use or if you have existing prostate conditions.

Caution:

- **Medications:** May interact with blood-thinning medications or hormone therapies. Consult a healthcare professional before use.
- **Pregnancy:** Avoid during pregnancy or while breastfeeding.

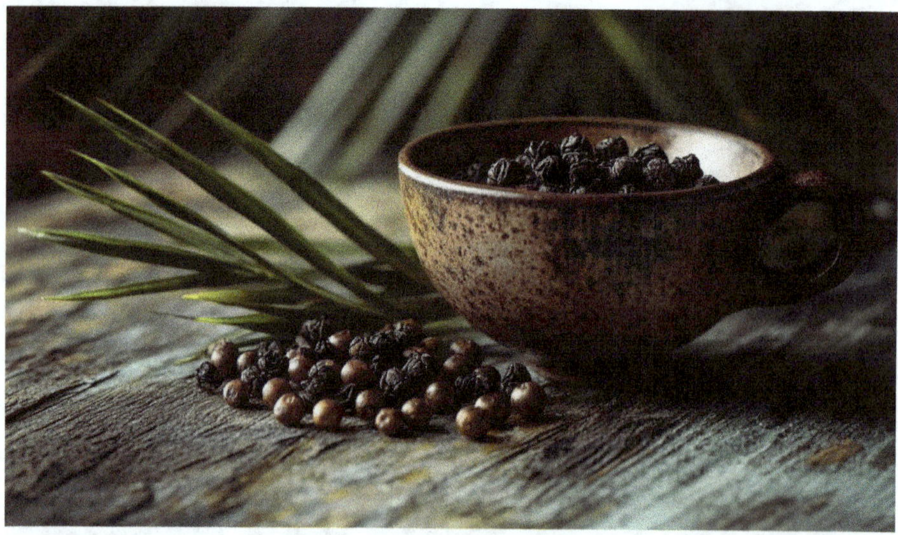

Recipe 32: Ginseng Energy Enhancement Elixir

Known as the "King of Herbs," ginseng has been revered for centuries in traditional Chinese medicine as a powerful adaptogen that boosts energy, reduces stress, and enhances stamina. This elixir combines ginseng with honey and lemon for a refreshing and revitalizing tonic, perfect for those seeking a natural energy boost.

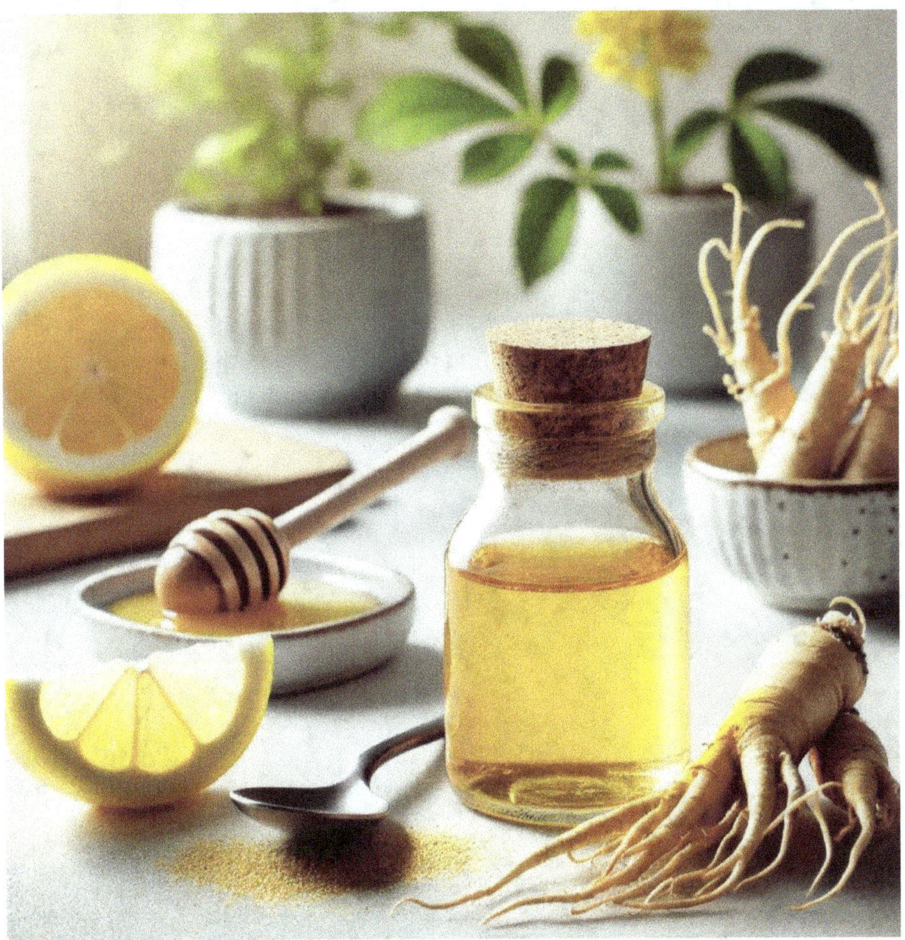

Ingredients:

- 1 teaspoon dried ginseng root or 1 small fresh root, sliced
- 1 cup water
- 1 tablespoon honey
- Juice of half a lemon

1. In a small saucepan, combine ginseng root and water.
2. Bring to a boil, then reduce heat and simmer for 15–20 minutes.
3. Remove from heat and strain the liquid into a cup.
4. Stir in honey and lemon juice.
5. Allow the elixir to cool slightly before drinking.

Usage:

- Drink one cup in the morning or early afternoon for sustained energy and focus.
- Avoid consuming late in the day to prevent difficulty sleeping.

Caution:

- **Medications:** Consult a healthcare provider if you are taking medications for diabetes, blood pressure, or mental health conditions.
- **Side Effects:** May cause restlessness or insomnia if taken in excess.

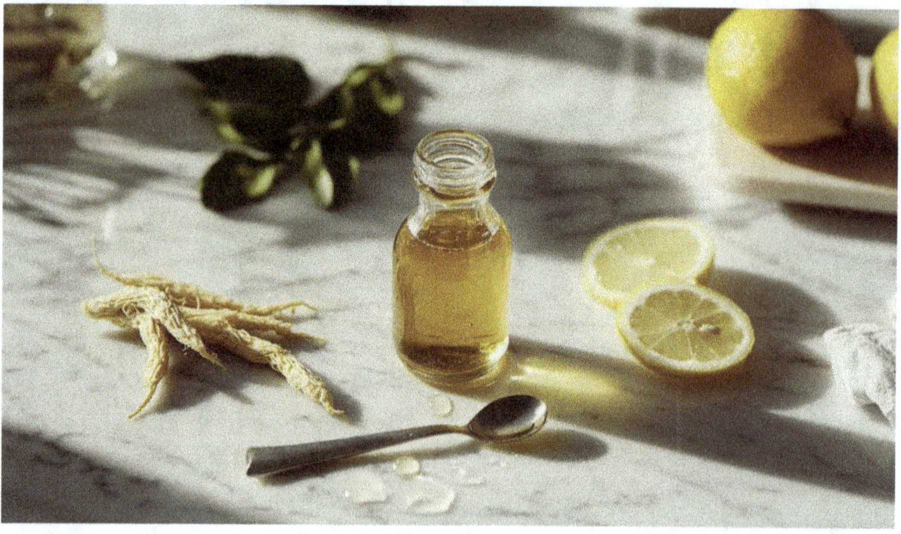

Recipe 33: Nettle Root Urinary Support Infusion

Nettle root, an ancient remedy in European folk medicine, is celebrated for its ability to support urinary tract function and prostate health. Its natural diuretic properties help flush toxins and reduce inflammation, making it an excellent herb for overall urinary health. This simple infusion is a convenient way to incorporate nettle root into daily life.

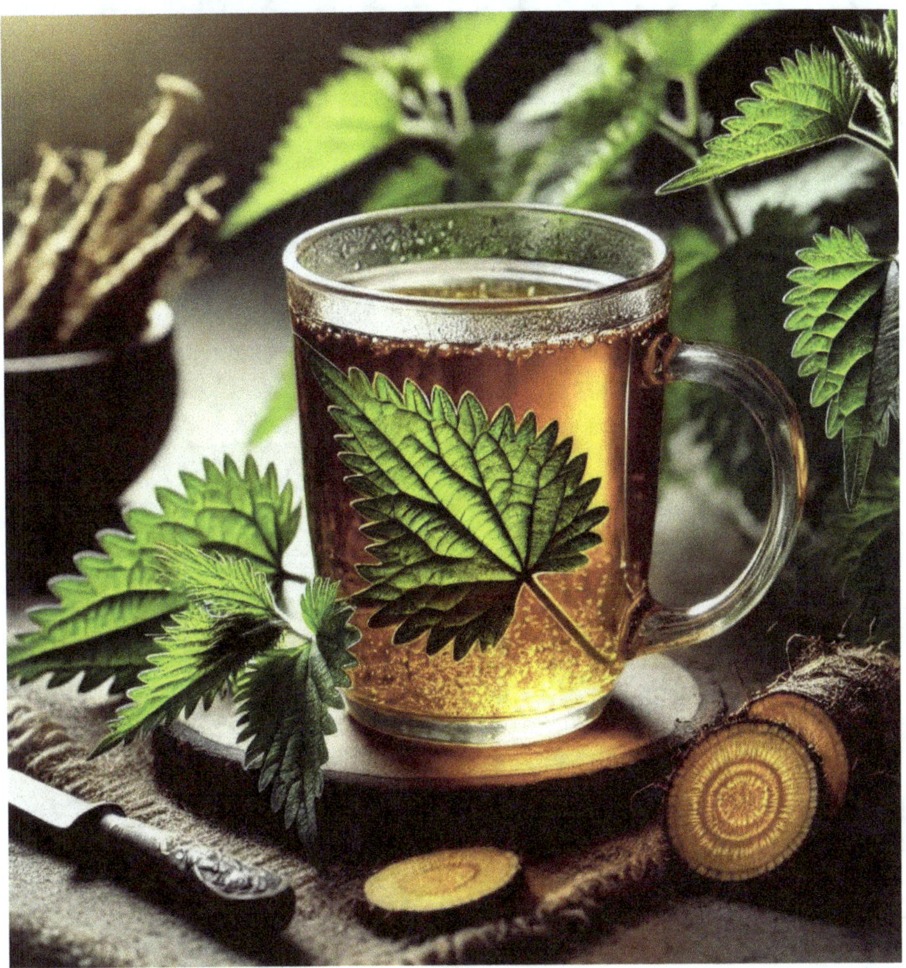

Ingredients:

- 1 tablespoon dried nettle root
- 1 cup boiling water
- Optional: Honey for sweetness

1. Place the dried nettle root in a teapot or infuser.
2. Pour boiling water over the root.
3. Cover and steep for 10–15 minutes.
4. Strain the tea into a cup.
5. Sweeten with honey if desired.

- Drink one to two cups daily to support urinary health and prostate function.
- Best consumed in the morning or afternoon.

- **Allergies:** Avoid if allergic to nettle or related plants.
- **Medications:** Consult a healthcare provider if taking diuretics or blood pressure medications.

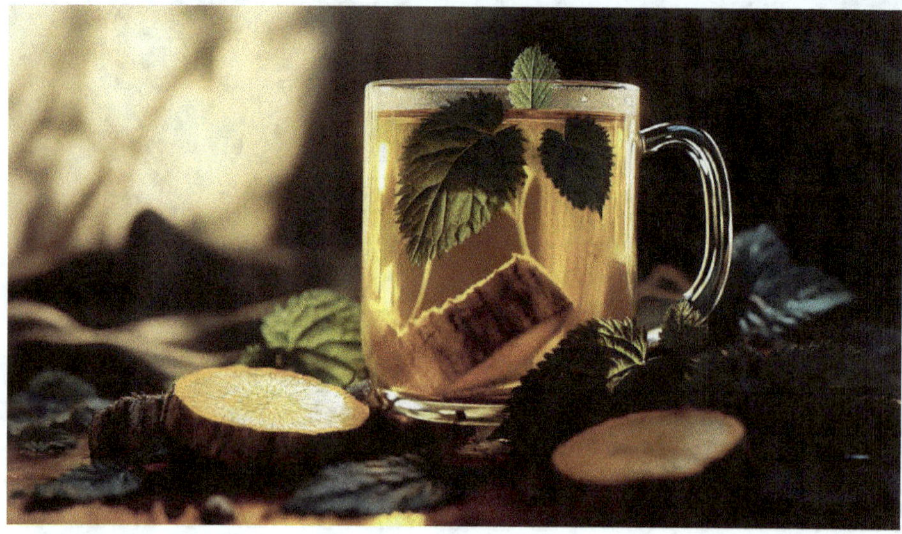

Recipe 34: Horny Goat Weed Vitality Tonic

Horny goat weed (*Epimedium*), a staple in traditional Chinese medicine, is widely known for its ability to support male vitality and stamina. This herbal tonic blends horny goat weed with cinnamon and honey, creating a warming and invigorating drink to enhance energy and overall well-being.

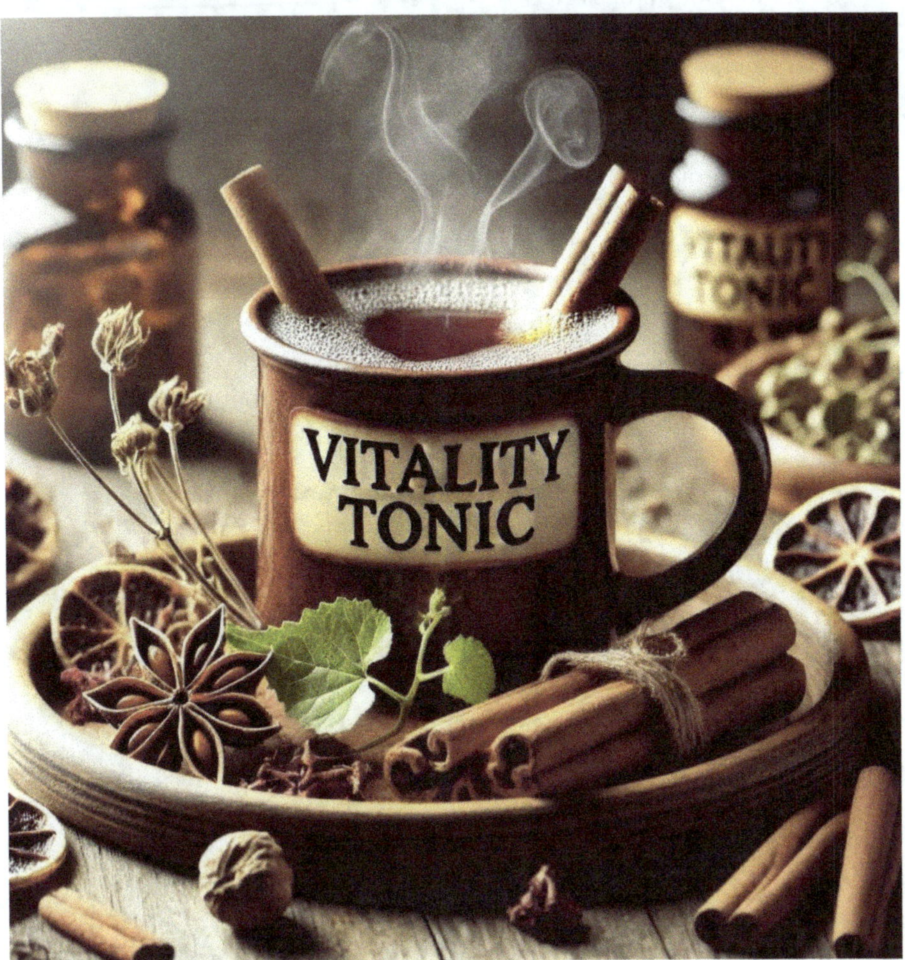

Ingredients:

- 1 teaspoon dried horny goat weed leaves
- 1 cinnamon stick
- 1 cup boiling water
- 1 teaspoon honey (optional)

1. Place horny goat weed leaves and the cinnamon stick in a teapot.
2. Pour boiling water over the herbs.
3. Cover and steep for 10 minutes.
4. Strain the liquid into a cup.
5. Stir in honey if desired.

Usage:

- Drink one cup daily to promote energy and vitality.
- Avoid prolonged use; take breaks after two to three weeks of consistent use.

Caution:

- **Medications:** May interact with medications for blood pressure or heart conditions. Consult a healthcare provider before use.
- **Side Effects:** High doses may cause dizziness or nausea.

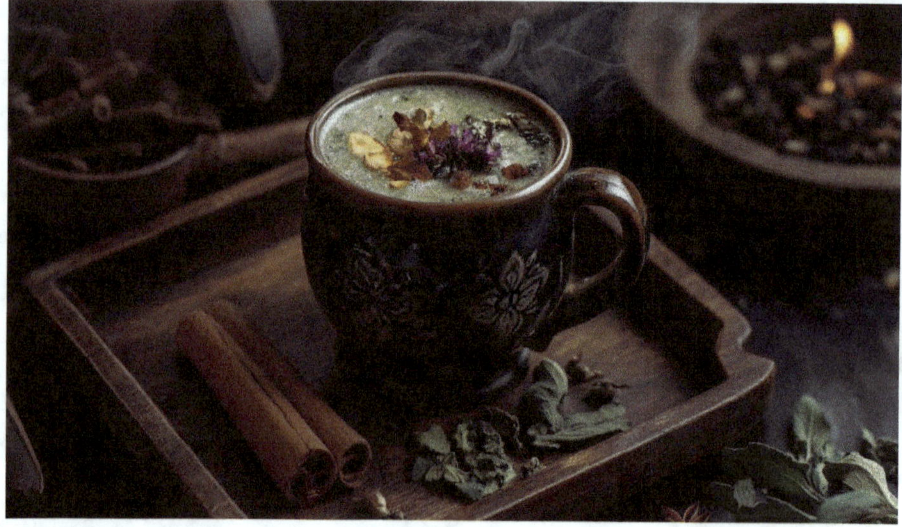

Recipe 35: Pumpkin Seed Oil Capsules for Wellness

Pumpkin seeds, rich in zinc and essential fatty acids, have long been valued for their role in supporting prostate health and overall wellness. Extracting the oil from these nutrient-dense seeds concentrates their benefits into a convenient and effective supplement. Pumpkin seed oil capsules are an easy addition to a daily wellness routine.

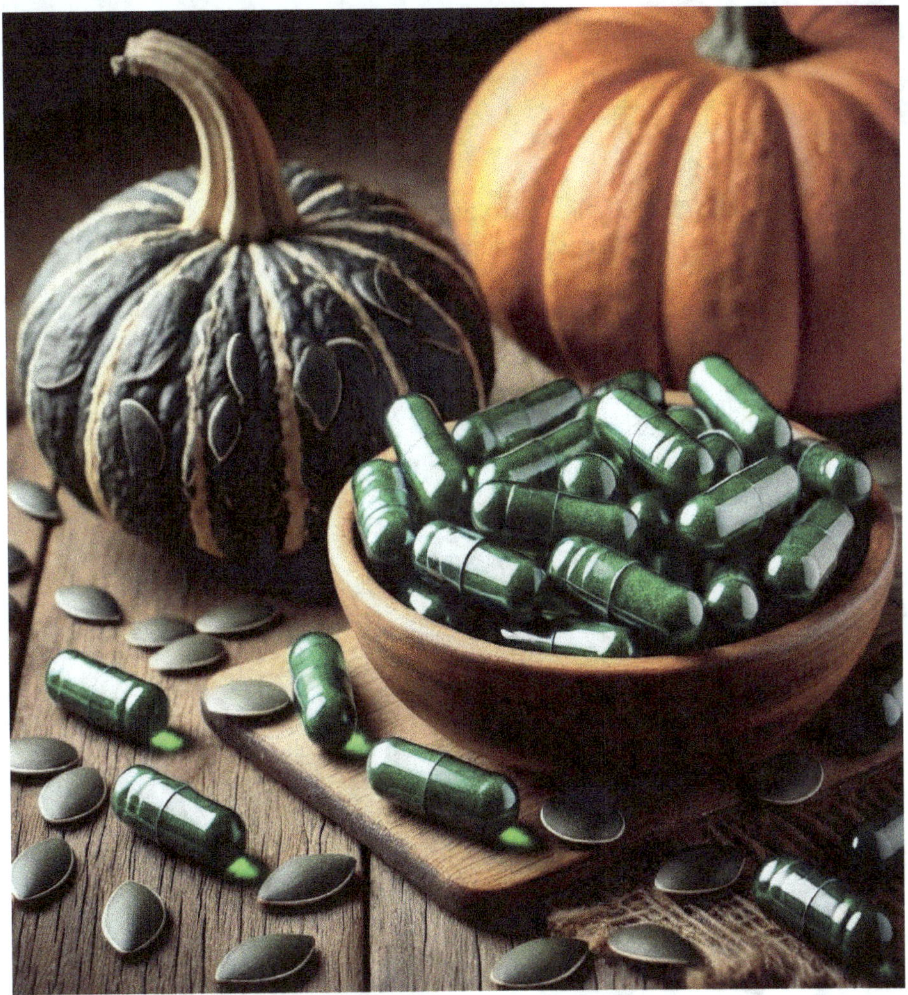

Ingredients:

- High-quality pumpkin seed oil capsules (500 mg or as directed on the packaging)

1. Purchase capsules from a trusted source.
2. Follow the dosage instructions on the label or as advised by a healthcare professional.

Usage:

- Take 1–2 capsules daily with meals to support prostate health and overall vitality.

Caution:

- **Allergies:** Avoid if allergic to pumpkin or related seeds.
- **Pregnancy and Breastfeeding:** Consult a healthcare provider before use.

Note: The remedies in this chapter are tailored to support men's health and well-being through natural ingredients and holistic practices. They are not substitutes for medical advice or treatment. Always consult a healthcare professional before starting a new supplement or herbal regimen, particularly if you have underlying health conditions or are taking medications.

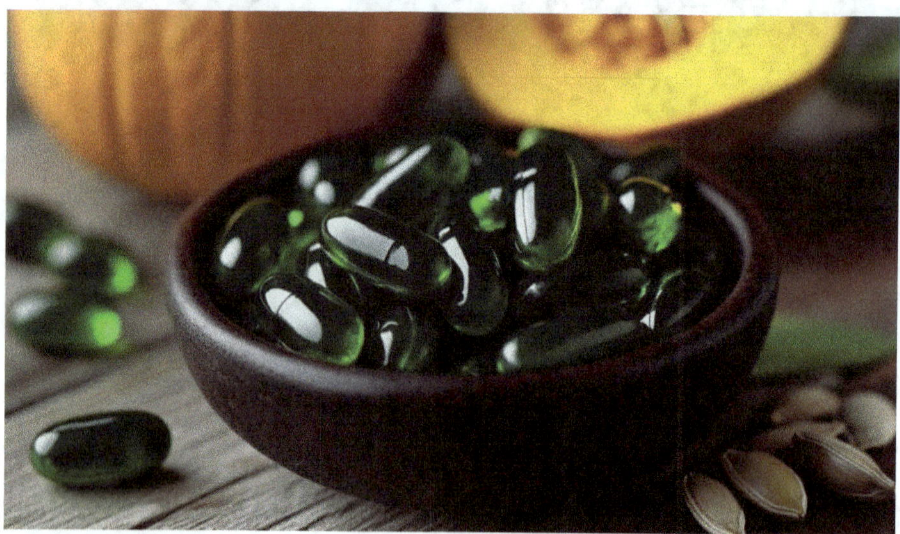

Recipe 36: Hawthorn Berry Heart Health Tea

Hawthorn berries have been a symbol of heart health since ancient times, used by herbalists to strengthen cardiovascular function and improve circulation. Rich in antioxidants like flavonoids and oligomeric procyanidins, these small red berries may help dilate blood vessels, improve blood flow, and reduce blood pressure. A warm cup of hawthorn berry tea is a comforting way to support your heart naturally.

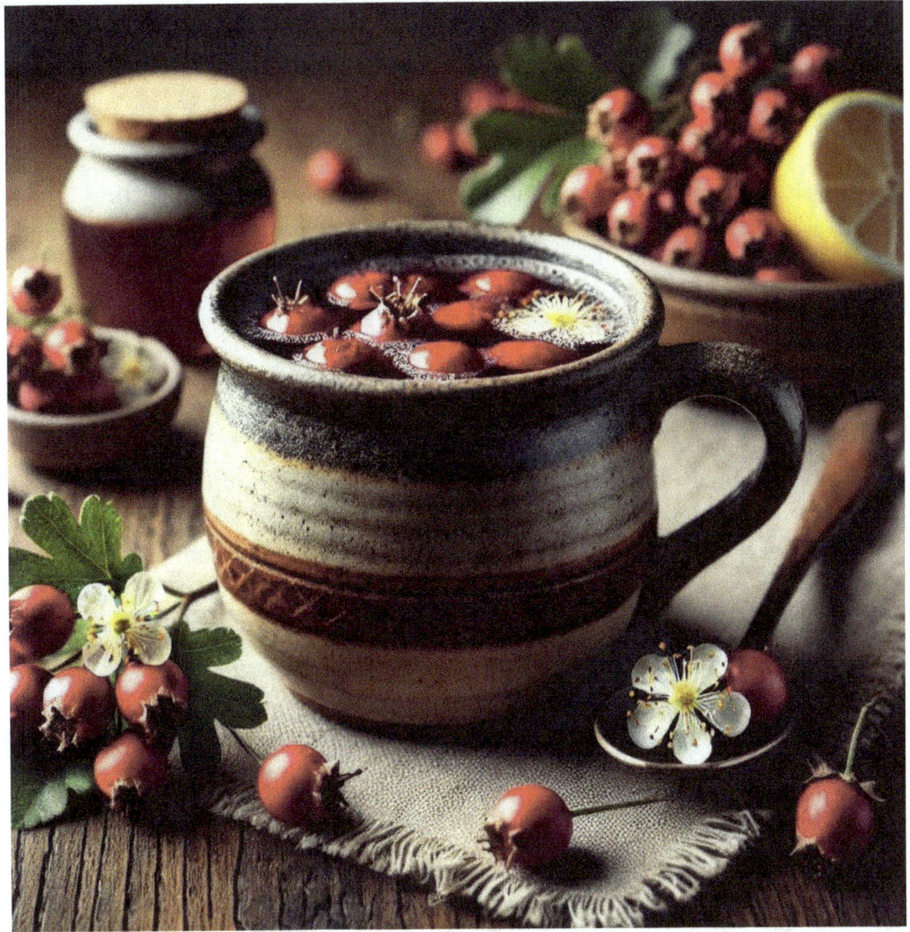

Ingredients:

- 1 tablespoon dried hawthorn berries
- 1 teaspoon dried hawthorn leaves and flowers (optional)

- 2 cups water
- Honey or lemon to taste (optional)

Instructions:

1. In a small saucepan, combine the dried hawthorn berries (and leaves and flowers if using) with water.
2. Bring to a gentle boil over medium heat.
3. Reduce heat and simmer for 10–15 minutes.
4. Remove from heat and let steep for an additional 10 minutes.
5. Strain the tea into a cup or teapot.
6. Add honey or lemon if desired.
7. Enjoy warm.

Usage:

- Drink one to two cups daily to support cardiovascular health.
- Consistent use over several weeks may yield the best results.

Caution:

- **Medications:** Consult a healthcare provider if you are taking heart medications, blood pressure drugs, or other cardiovascular treatments.
- **Pregnancy and Breastfeeding:** Not recommended without professional guidance.
- **Allergies:** Avoid if allergic to plants in the Rosaceae family.

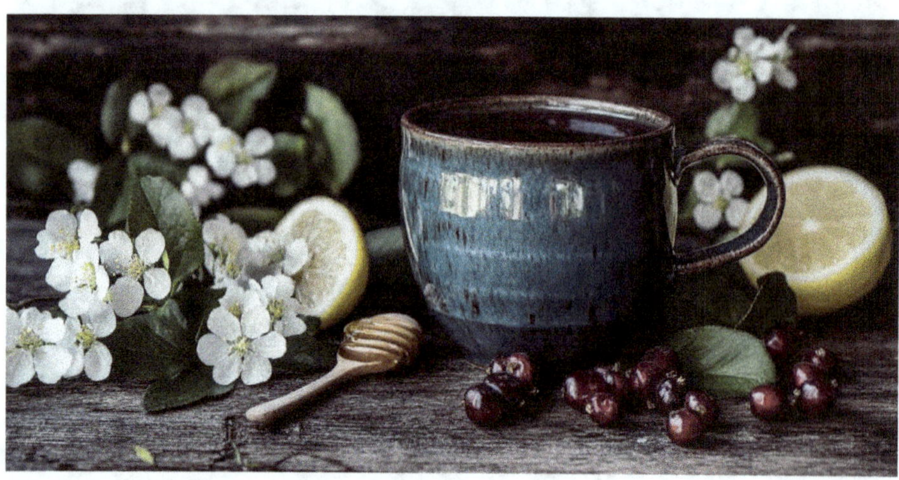

Recipe 37: Ginkgo Biloba Circulation Boosting Infusion

Ginkgo biloba, one of the oldest living tree species, has been used in traditional Chinese medicine for thousands of years. Known for its potential to improve blood flow and enhance cognitive function, ginkgo may help with memory, focus, and circulation issues. This light and refreshing infusion is a simple way to incorporate ginkgo's benefits into your daily routine.

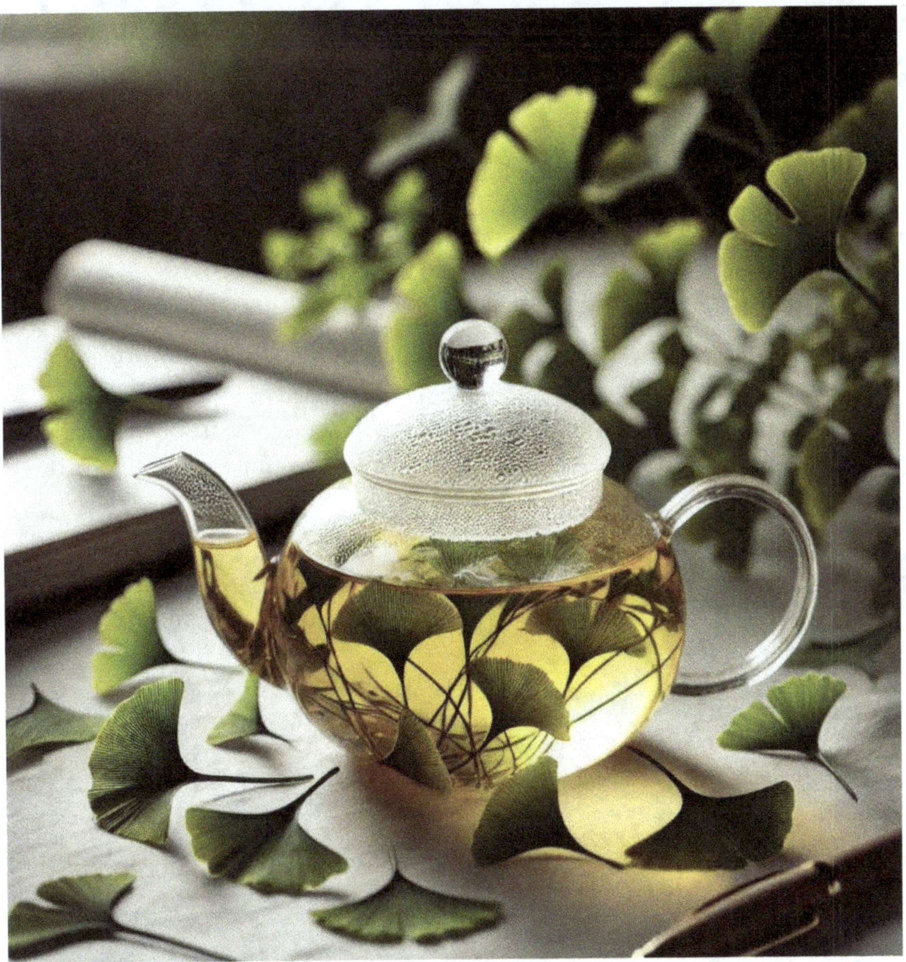

Ingredients:

- 1 teaspoon dried ginkgo biloba leaves
- 1 cup boiling water
- Honey or lemon (optional)

1. Place the dried ginkgo leaves in a tea infuser or teapot.
2. Pour boiling water over the leaves.
3. Cover and let steep for 5–10 minutes.
4. Strain the infusion into a cup.
5. Add honey or lemon if desired.
6. Enjoy warm.

Usage:

- Drink one cup daily to support circulation and cognitive function.
- Morning consumption is ideal to promote alertness throughout the day.

Caution:

- **Medications:** May interact with blood thinners, antidepressants, and anti-seizure drugs. Consult a healthcare provider before use.
- **Side Effects:** Possible mild gastrointestinal discomfort or headache.
- **Pregnancy and Breastfeeding:** Avoid use unless directed by a professional.

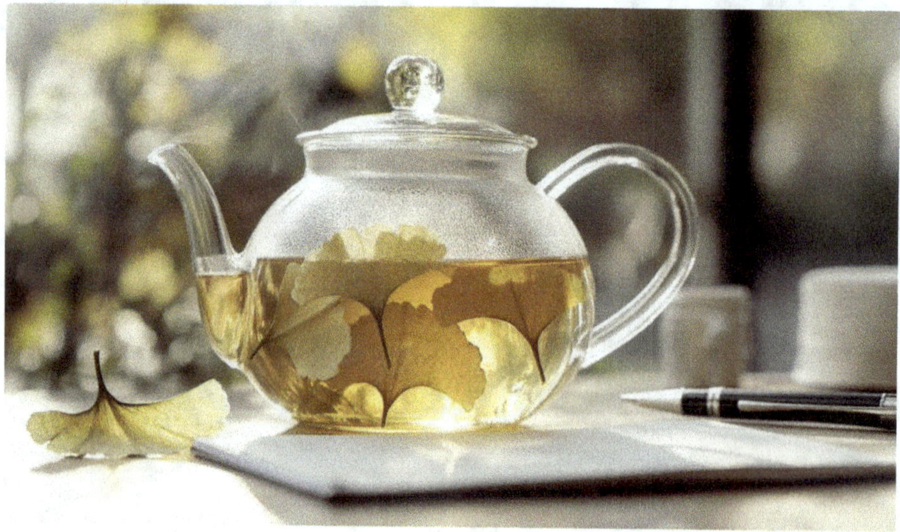

Recipe 38: Cayenne Pepper Circulatory Stimulating Tincture

Cayenne pepper, derived from hot chili peppers, is famed for its ability to stimulate circulation and warm the body. Capsaicin, the active component, may help strengthen the heart, regulate blood flow, and reduce cholesterol levels. A tincture made from cayenne offers a potent and convenient way to harness these fiery benefits.

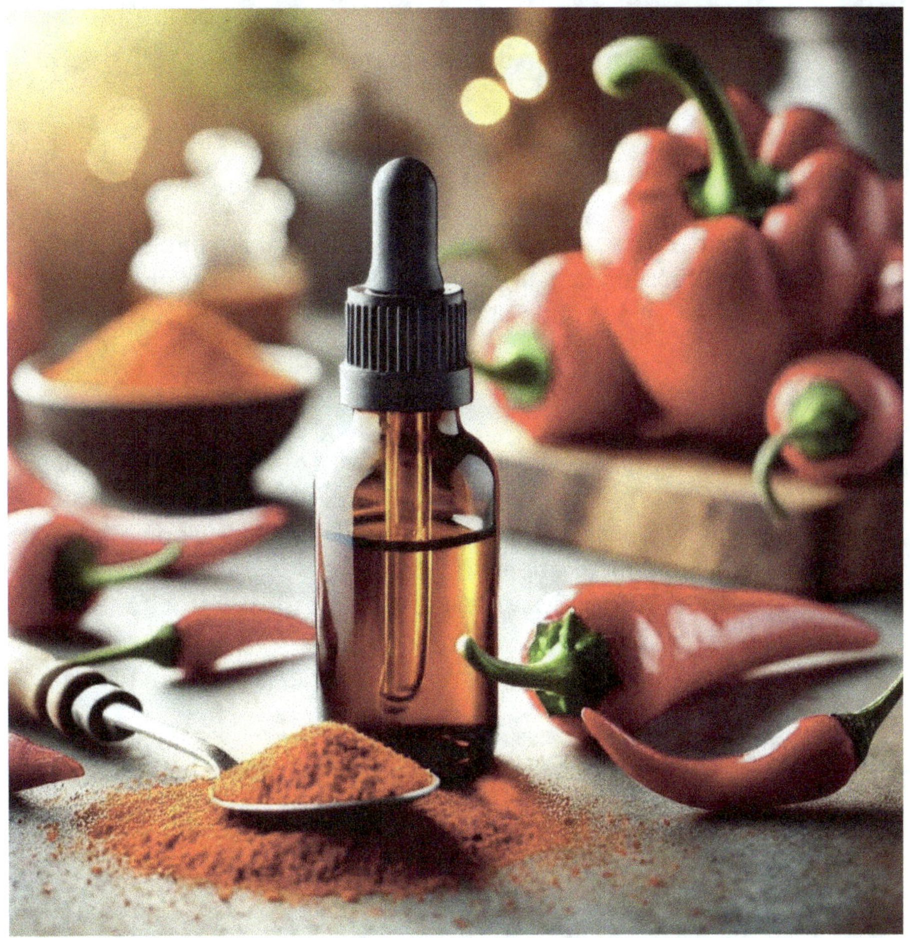

Ingredients:

- ¼ cup cayenne pepper powder (30,000–50,000 Scoville heat units)
- 1 cup vodka or apple cider vinegar (for alcohol-free option)
- Glass jar with tight-fitting lid
- Dropper bottles for storage

Instructions:

1. Place cayenne pepper powder in the glass jar.
2. Pour vodka or apple cider vinegar over the powder, ensuring it's fully covered.
3. Seal the jar tightly and shake well.
4. Store in a cool, dark place for 2–4 weeks, shaking daily.
5. After steeping, strain the liquid through a fine mesh strainer or cheesecloth into a bowl.
6. Transfer the tincture into dropper bottles.
7. Label and date the bottles.

Usage:

- Start with 5–10 drops diluted in water or juice, up to three times daily.
- Can be increased gradually to 20–30 drops if well-tolerated.
- Take before meals to stimulate digestion and circulation.

Caution:

- **Spiciness:** Cayenne is very hot; handle with care to avoid skin and eye irritation.
- **Medications:** Consult a healthcare provider if taking blood thinners or blood pressure medications.
- **Stomach Sensitivity:** May cause gastrointestinal discomfort; do not take on an empty stomach.
- **Pregnancy and Breastfeeding:** Use only under professional guidance.

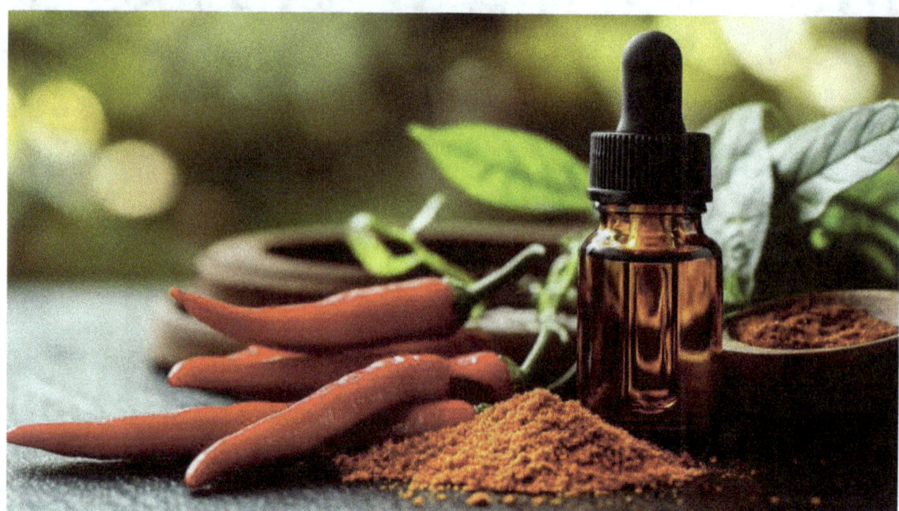

Recipe 39: Ginger and Garlic Cardiovascular Support Mix

Ginger and garlic, staples in kitchens worldwide, are more than just flavorful ingredients—they're powerful allies for heart health. Ginger aids in improving circulation and reducing inflammation, while garlic is known for lowering cholesterol and blood pressure. Together, they form a potent mix to support cardiovascular wellness.

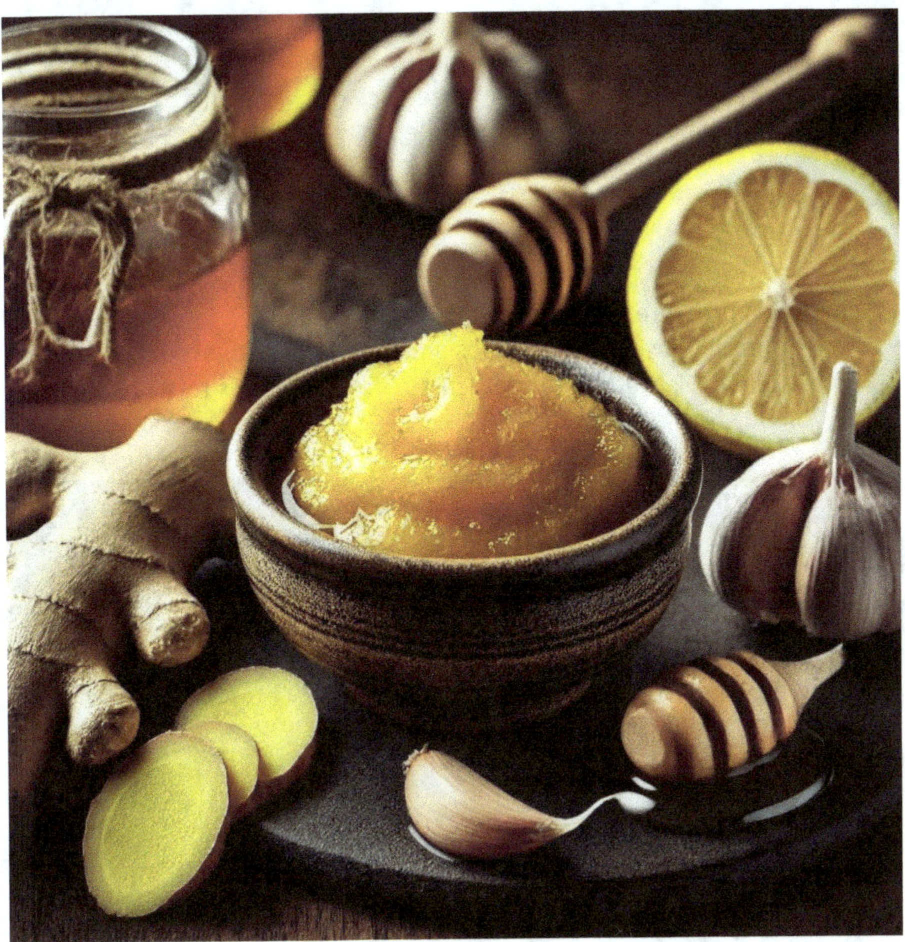

Ingredients:

- 2 tablespoons fresh ginger root, grated
- 2 tablespoons fresh garlic cloves, minced
- ¼ cup raw honey
- Juice of one lemon (optional)

1. In a clean bowl, combine grated ginger and minced garlic.
2. Add raw honey and mix thoroughly to form a paste.
3. Stir in lemon juice if desired.
4. Transfer the mixture to a glass jar with a lid.
5. Store in the refrigerator for up to one week.

Usage:

- Take one teaspoon of the mixture once or twice daily.
- Can be consumed directly or diluted in warm water as a tea.

Caution:

- **Medications:** Consult a healthcare provider if taking anticoagulants, blood pressure, or diabetes medications.
- **Stomach Sensitivity:** May cause mild gastrointestinal discomfort.
- **Surgery:** Discontinue use at least two weeks prior to surgery due to blood-thinning effects.

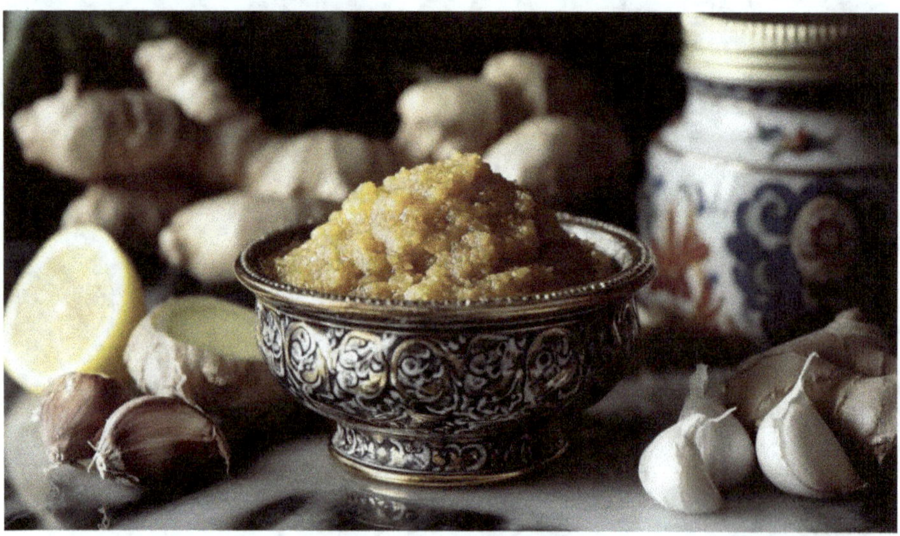

Recipe 40: Bilberry Eye Health Decoction

Bilberries, closely related to blueberries, are rich in anthocyanins—antioxidants that support vascular health and improve circulation, particularly in the tiny capillaries of the eyes. Traditionally used to enhance night vision and reduce eye fatigue, bilberry may also benefit overall circulatory function.

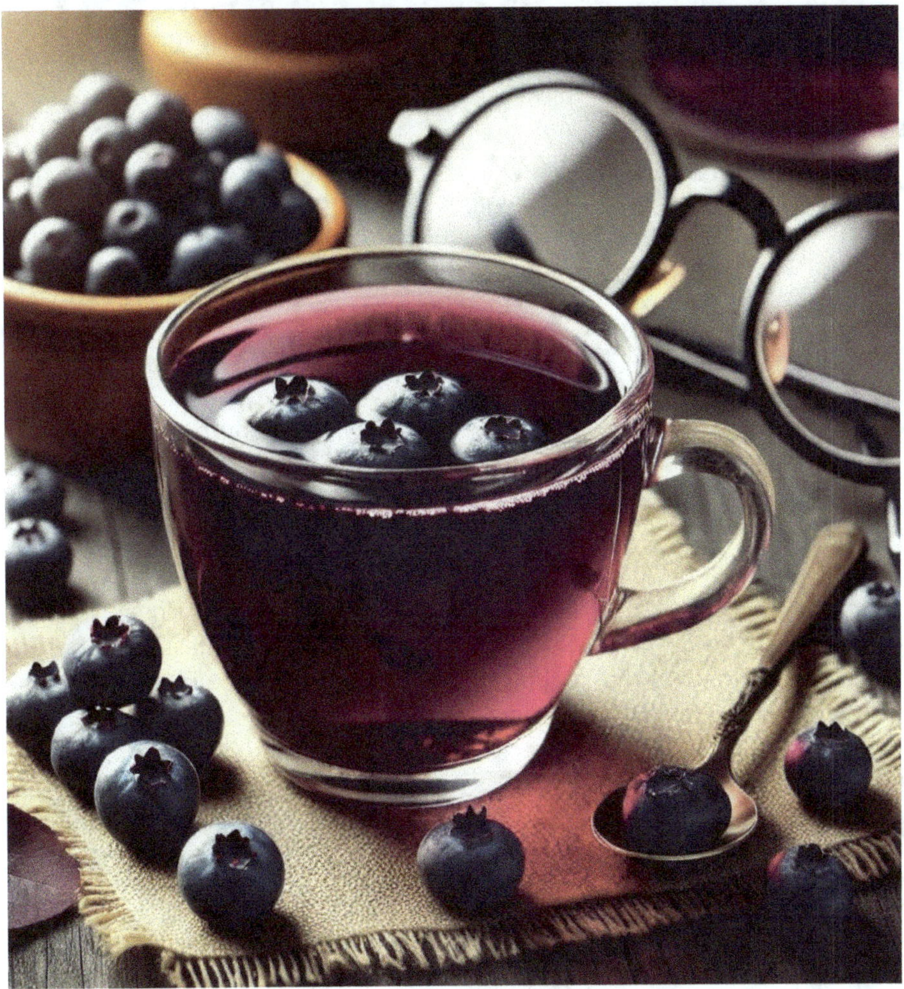

Ingredients:

- 2 tablespoons dried bilberries
- 2 cups water
- Honey to taste (optional)

1. Combine dried bilberries and water in a saucepan.
2. Bring to a boil over medium heat.
3. Reduce heat and simmer for 20 minutes.
4. Remove from heat and let cool slightly.
5. Strain the liquid into a cup or teapot.
6. Sweeten with honey if desired.

Usage:

- Drink one cup daily to support eye and circulatory health.
- Can be enjoyed warm or chilled.

Caution:

- **Medications:** Consult a healthcare provider if taking blood sugar-lowering medications.
- **Allergies:** Avoid if allergic to bilberries or similar berries.
- **Pregnancy and Breastfeeding:** Safety not well-established; consult a professional before use.

Note: The herbal remedies provided in this chapter are intended to support circulatory health and are not replacements for professional medical treatment. Always consult a qualified healthcare professional before beginning any new herbal regimen, especially if you have underlying health conditions or are taking medications.

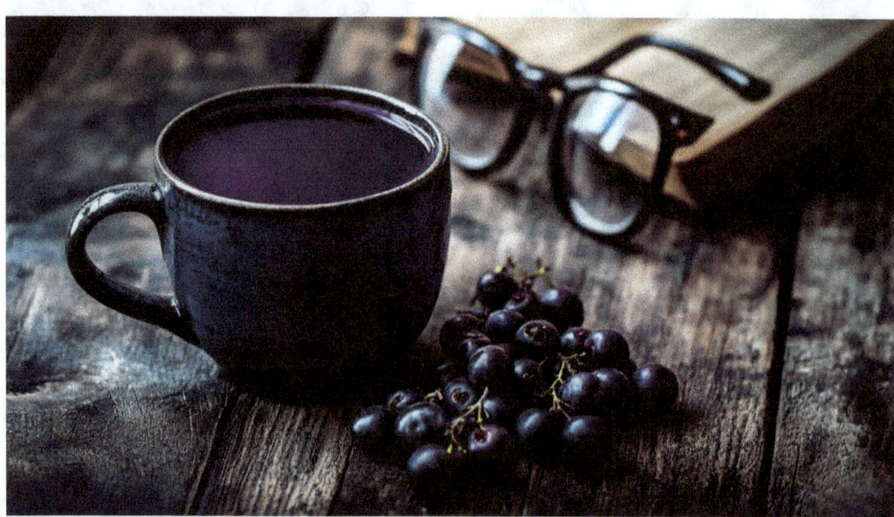

Recipe 41: White Willow Bark Headache Tea

Long before the advent of modern pain relievers, white willow bark was a go-to remedy for aches and fevers. Containing salicin, a natural compound similar to aspirin's active ingredient, white willow bark has been used for millennia to alleviate headaches and reduce inflammation. This gentle tea offers a natural alternative for those seeking relief from occasional discomfort.

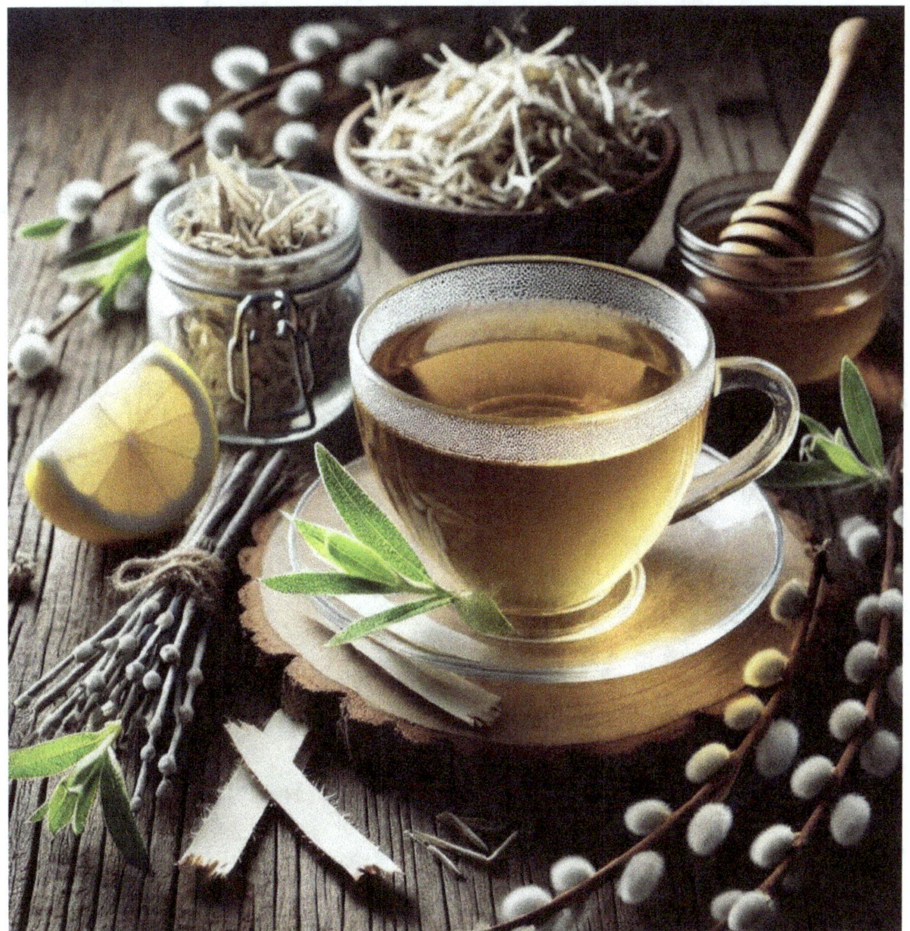

Ingredients:

- 2 teaspoons dried white willow bark
- 1 cup boiling water
- Honey or lemon (optional)

1. Place the dried white willow bark in a small saucepan.
2. Add boiling water and bring to a simmer over low heat.
3. Simmer gently for 10–15 minutes to extract the beneficial compounds.
4. Remove from heat and let steep for an additional 5 minutes.
5. Strain the tea into a cup using a fine mesh strainer.
6. Add honey or lemon if desired.
7. Sip slowly and relax.

Usage:

- Drink one cup up to twice daily for relief from mild headaches and general aches.

Caution:

- **Allergies:** Avoid if allergic to aspirin or salicylates.
- **Medical Conditions:** Not recommended for individuals with asthma, bleeding disorders, or gastrointestinal ulcers.
- **Medications:** Consult a healthcare provider if taking anticoagulants or other medications.
- **Pregnancy and Breastfeeding:** Not advised during pregnancy or breastfeeding.

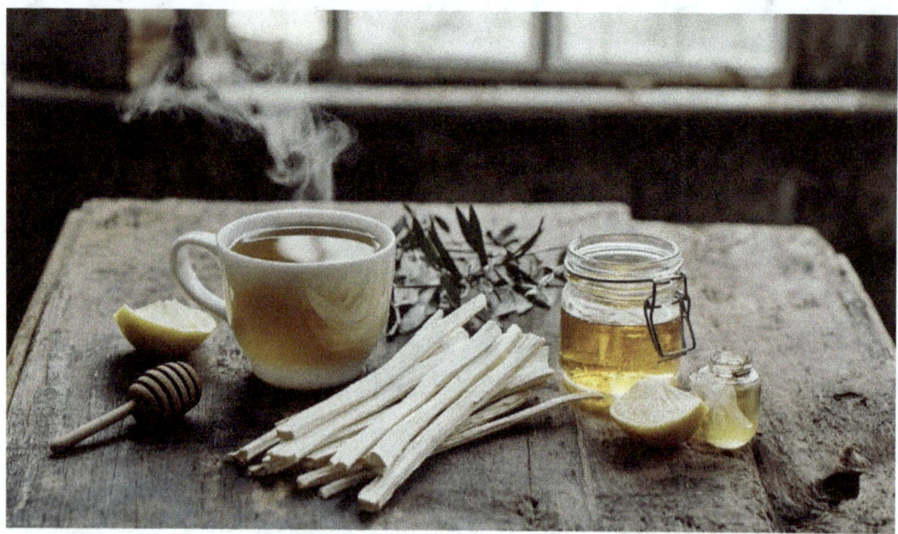

Recipe 42: Arnica Muscle Ache Salve

Arnica, a bright yellow mountain flower, has been treasured for centuries for its ability to soothe sore muscles, bruises, and sprains. Its anti-inflammatory and analgesic properties make it a staple in herbal first aid kits. Creating a topical salve with arnica allows for targeted relief of muscle discomfort and promotes healing.

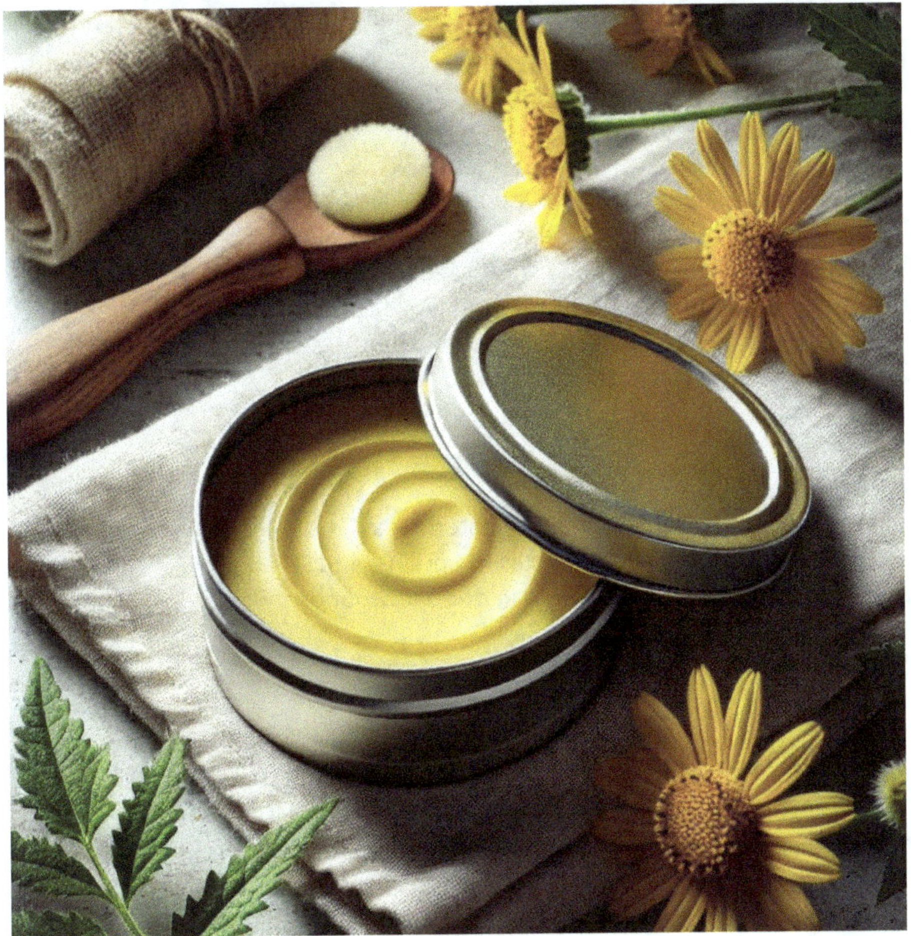

Ingredients:

- 1 cup carrier oil (e.g., olive oil or sweet almond oil)
- ½ cup dried arnica flowers
- ¼ cup beeswax pellets
- Optional: 10 drops lavender essential oil for added soothing effect
- Sterilized jars or tins for storage

Instructions:

Infuse the Oil:

1. Combine dried arnica flowers and carrier oil in a glass jar.
2. Seal the jar and place it in a sunny spot for 4–6 weeks, shaking occasionally. For a quicker method, gently heat the mixture in a double boiler for 2 hours on low heat.
3. Strain the infused oil through cheesecloth into a clean bowl, pressing to extract all the oil.

Make the Salve:

4. In a double boiler, combine the arnica-infused oil and beeswax.
5. Heat gently until the beeswax melts completely.
6. Remove from heat and stir in lavender essential oil if using.
7. Pour the mixture into sterilized jars or tins.
8. Allow the salve to cool and solidify before sealing.
9. Label and date your containers.

Usage:

- Apply a small amount to affected areas 2–3 times daily.
- Use for muscle aches, bruises, sprains, and swelling.
- Do not apply to broken skin or open wounds.

Caution:

- **External Use Only:** Do not ingest arnica; it's toxic when taken internally.
- **Skin Sensitivity:** Perform a patch test to check for allergic reactions.
- **Pregnancy and Breastfeeding:** Consult a healthcare professional before use.

Recipe 43: Devil's Claw Joint Pain Relief Tea

Native to the arid regions of southern Africa, devil's claw is named for its distinctive hooked fruit. Traditionally used by the indigenous people to treat pain and inflammation, this herb is renowned for its potential to ease joint discomfort associated with arthritis and rheumatism. A warm cup of devil's claw tea may offer natural relief for stiff or achy joints.

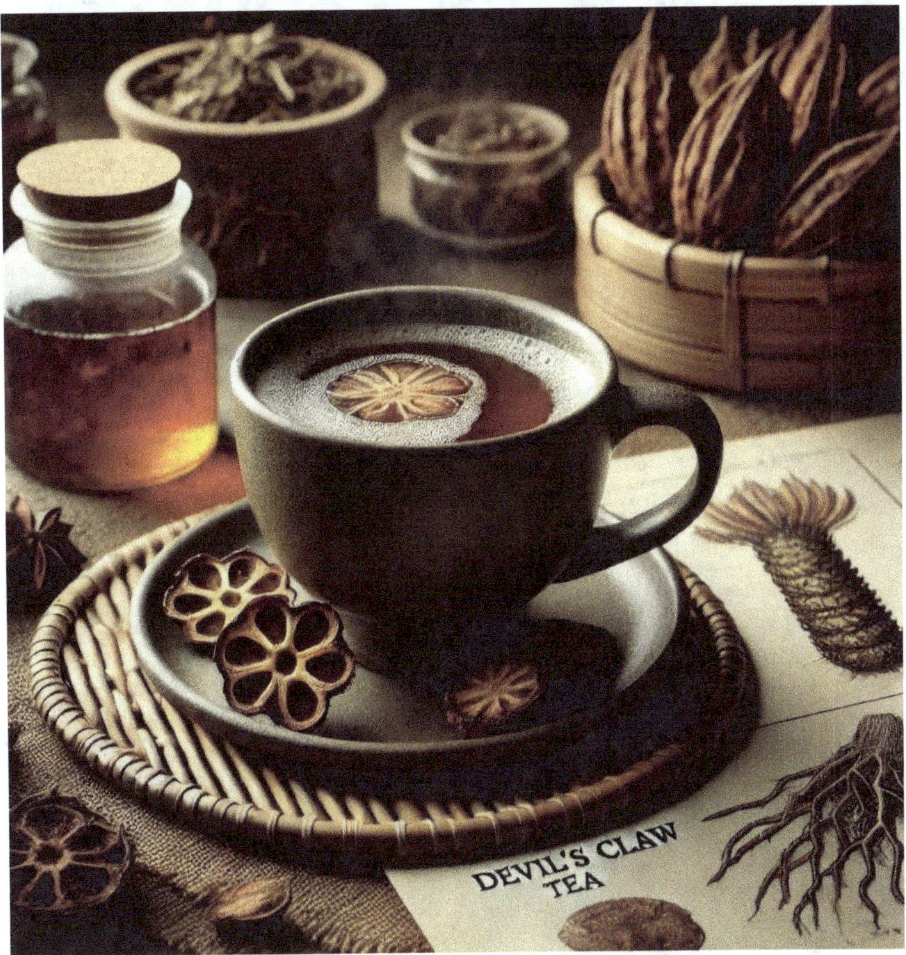

Ingredients:

- 1 teaspoon dried devil's claw root
- 1 cup water
- Honey or cinnamon (optional, to improve taste)

1. In a small saucepan, combine the dried devil's claw root and water.
2. Bring to a boil over medium heat.
3. Reduce heat and simmer for 15 minutes.
4. Remove from heat and let steep for an additional 5 minutes.
5. Strain the tea into a cup.
6. Add honey or a pinch of cinnamon to enhance flavor if desired.
7. Enjoy warm.

- Drink one cup up to twice daily to help alleviate joint pain.
- Consistent use over several weeks may provide the best results.

- **Medical Conditions:** Not recommended for individuals with stomach ulcers, gallstones, or heart conditions.
- **Medications:** Consult a healthcare provider if taking blood thinners or diabetes medications.
- **Pregnancy and Breastfeeding:** Avoid use during pregnancy and breastfeeding.

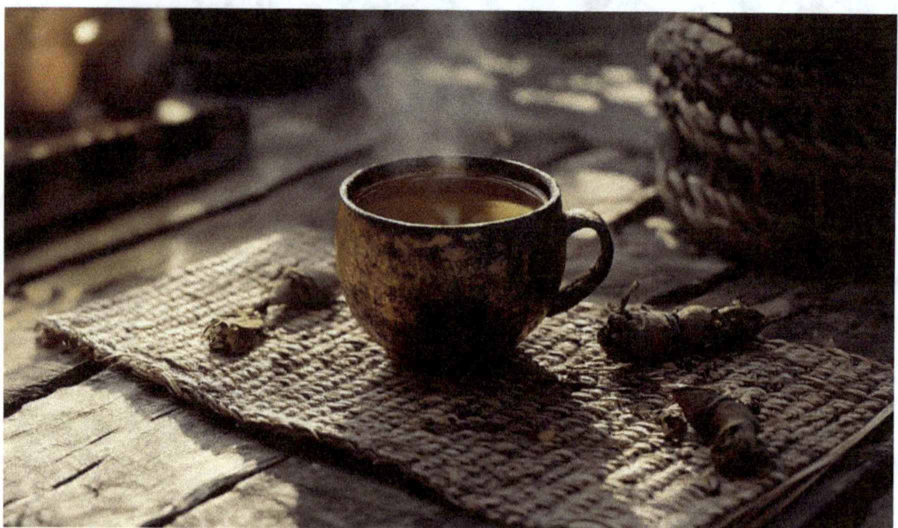

Recipe 44: St. John's Wort Nerve Pain Oil

St. John's Wort, with its bright yellow flowers, has been a beacon of healing since ancient times. While often recognized for its mood-lifting properties, it also possesses analgesic qualities that can help alleviate nerve pain, such as sciatica or shingles. Infusing oil with St. John's Wort creates a soothing topical remedy to ease discomfort and support nerve health.

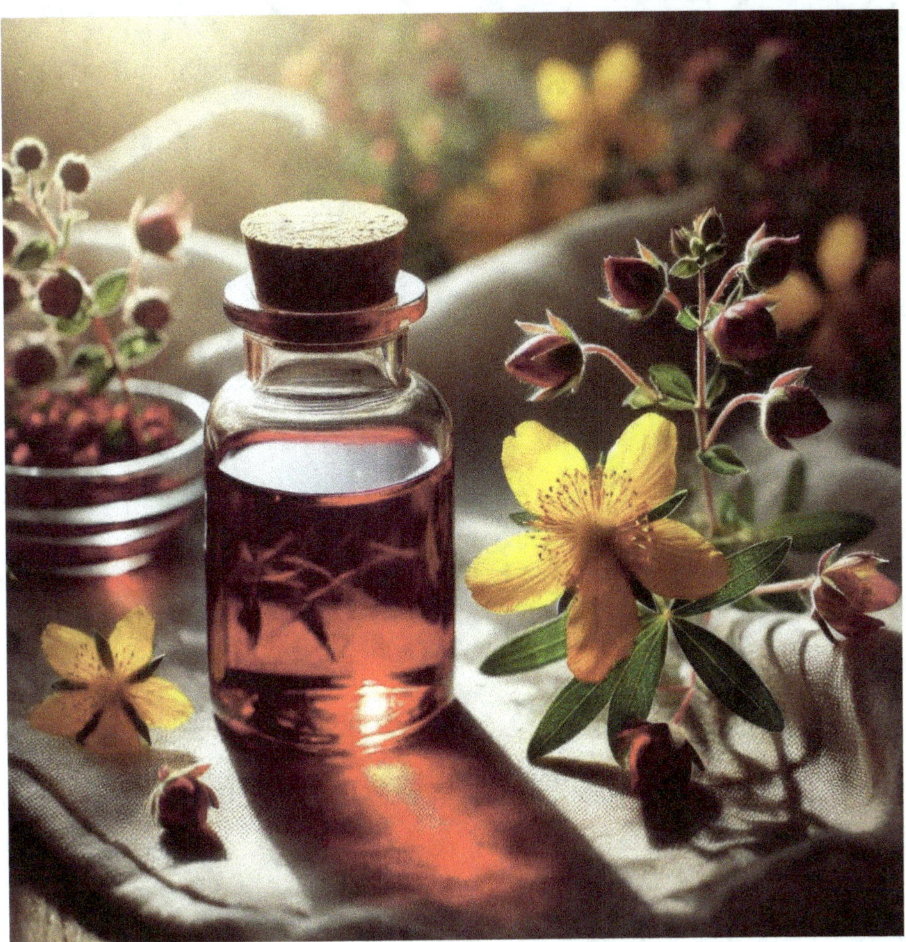

Ingredients:

- 1 cup fresh St. John's Wort flowers (or ½ cup dried)
- 1 cup carrier oil (e.g., olive oil or sweet almond oil)
- Clean glass jar with tight-fitting lid
- Cheesecloth or fine mesh strainer

1. Lightly crush the St. John's Wort flowers to release their oils.
2. Place the flowers in the glass jar.
3. Pour the carrier oil over the flowers, ensuring they are fully submerged.
4. Seal the jar and place it in a sunny spot for 4–6 weeks. The oil will turn a deep red color.
5. Shake the jar gently every few days.
6. After infusion, strain the oil through cheesecloth into a clean container.
7. Transfer the infused oil into a dark glass bottle for storage.
8. Label and date the bottle.

Usage:

- Gently massage a small amount of oil onto affected areas 2–3 times daily.
- Ideal for nerve pain, minor burns, and bruises.

Caution:

- **Sun Sensitivity:** St. John's Wort may increase skin sensitivity to sunlight. Avoid direct sun exposure on treated areas.
- **Medications:** Can interact with certain medications if absorbed systemically. Consult a healthcare provider if you are taking prescriptions.
- **Allergies:** Perform a patch test to check for skin sensitivity.

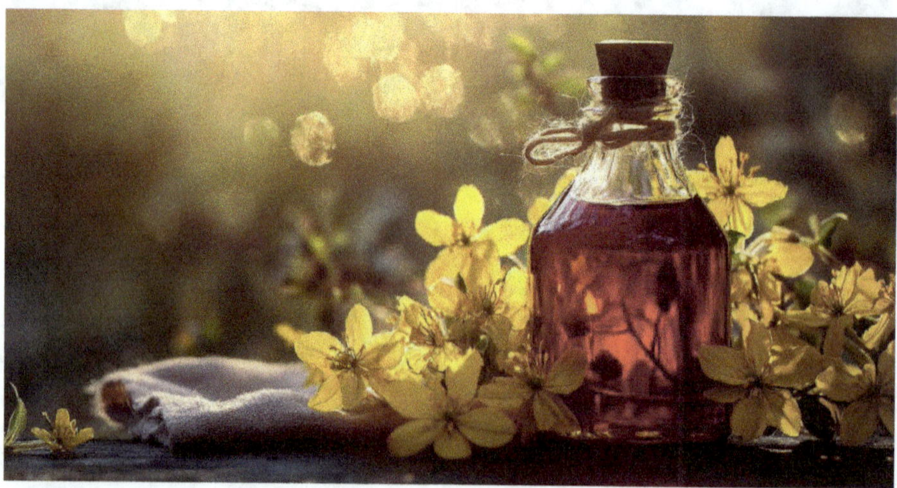

Recipe 45: Turmeric and Black Pepper Anti-Inflammatory Paste

Turmeric, the golden spice cherished in Ayurvedic medicine, is celebrated for its potent anti-inflammatory properties due to the compound curcumin. When combined with black pepper, which enhances curcumin's absorption, it becomes an even more powerful ally against inflammation and pain. This versatile paste can be used in cooking or stirred into warm beverages for a healthful boost.

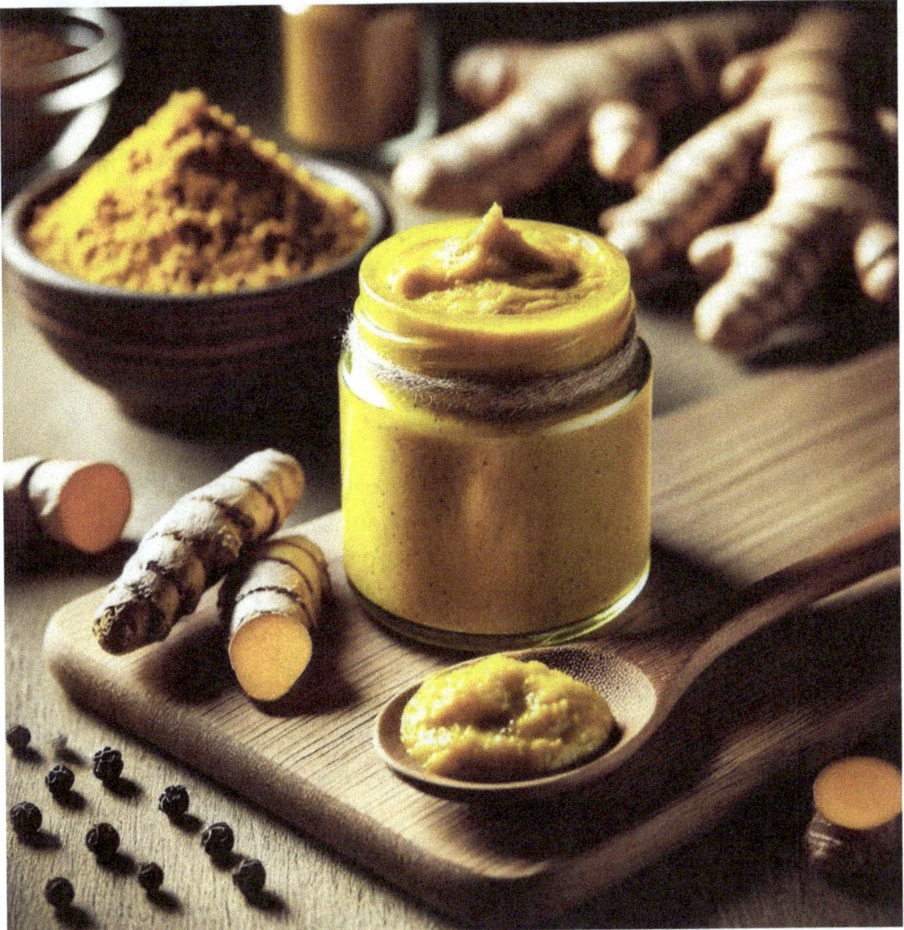

Ingredients:

- ½ cup turmeric powder
- 1 cup water (plus additional if needed)
- 1½ teaspoons ground black pepper
- 5 tablespoons extra virgin olive oil or coconut oil

1. In a small saucepan, combine turmeric powder and water over medium-low heat.
2. Stir continuously until a thick paste forms, about 7–10 minutes. Add more water if necessary.
3. Remove from heat and let cool slightly.
4. Stir in ground black pepper and oil until fully incorporated.
5. Transfer the paste into a sterilized glass jar with a lid.
6. Store in the refrigerator for up to two weeks.

Usage:

- **As a Beverage:** Stir 1 teaspoon of paste into a cup of warm milk (dairy or plant-based) for a soothing drink.
- **In Cooking:** Add to soups, stews, or rice dishes for flavor and health benefits.
- **Topical Application:** Mix with a small amount of water to create a paste and apply to sore joints (may stain skin and fabrics).

Caution:

- **Staining:** Turmeric can stain skin and clothing; handle with care.
- **Medical Conditions:** Consult a healthcare provider if you have gallbladder disease or are taking blood thinners.
- **Pregnancy and Breastfeeding:** Generally safe in food amounts, but consult a professional before using medicinal doses.

Note: The remedies in this chapter aim to provide natural support for occasional pain and discomfort. They are not a substitute for professional medical advice or treatment. Persistent or severe pain should be evaluated by a healthcare professional. Always consult a qualified provider before starting any new herbal regimen, especially if you have underlying health conditions or are taking medications.

Recipe 46: Maca Root Energizing Smoothie

High in the Andes Mountains of Peru, maca root has been cultivated for over 2,000 years. Revered as a superfood, maca is known for its potential to enhance energy, stamina, and endurance. Rich in vitamins, minerals, and amino acids, this adaptogenic root helps the body adapt to stress and supports overall vitality. Blending maca into a delicious smoothie is a convenient and tasty way to harness its energizing benefits.

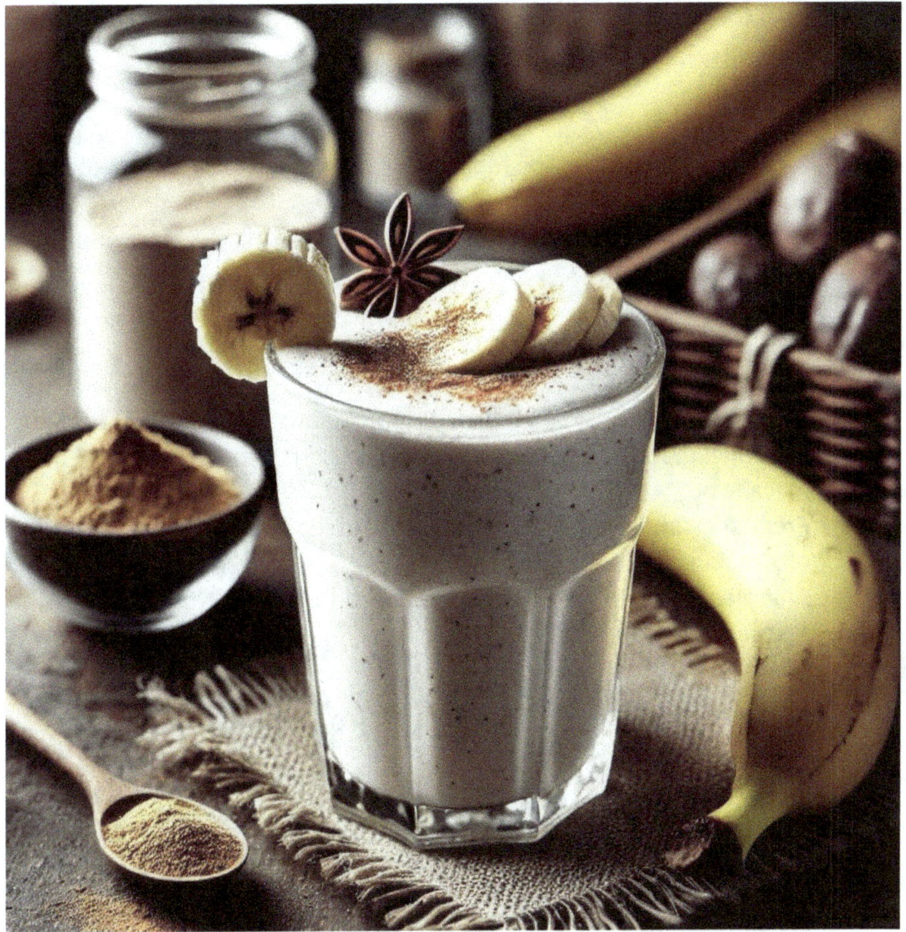

Ingredients:

- 1 ripe banana
- 1 cup almond milk (or milk of choice)

- 1 tablespoon maca root powder
- 1 teaspoon honey or maple syrup (optional, for sweetness)
- ½ teaspoon ground cinnamon
- A handful of ice cubes

Instructions:

1. Peel the banana and break it into chunks.
2. Place all ingredients into a blender.
3. Blend on high speed until smooth and creamy.
4. Taste and adjust sweetness if necessary.
5. Pour into a glass and enjoy immediately.

Usage:

- Enjoy this smoothie in the morning or as a midday pick-me-up to boost energy levels naturally.
- Incorporate it into your routine before workouts for enhanced stamina.

Caution:

- **Medical Conditions:** If you have thyroid issues or are taking hormone-sensitive medications, consult a healthcare provider before using maca root.
- **Pregnancy and Breastfeeding:** Limited research is available; consult a professional before use.
- **Allergies:** Monitor for any adverse reactions when trying maca for the first time.

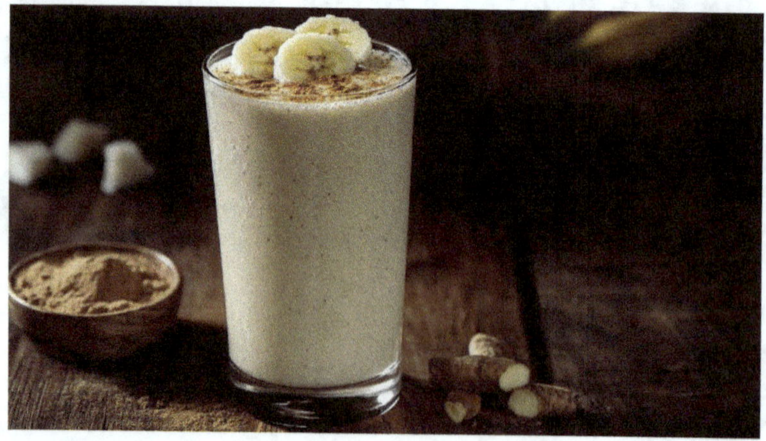

Recipe 47: Ashwagandha Stress Relief Tea

Ashwagandha, a prominent herb in Ayurvedic medicine, is celebrated for its ability to combat stress and promote relaxation while simultaneously boosting energy levels. Known as an adaptogen, it helps the body manage physical and mental stressors. This earthy tea provides a calming yet invigorating experience, supporting balance and vitality.

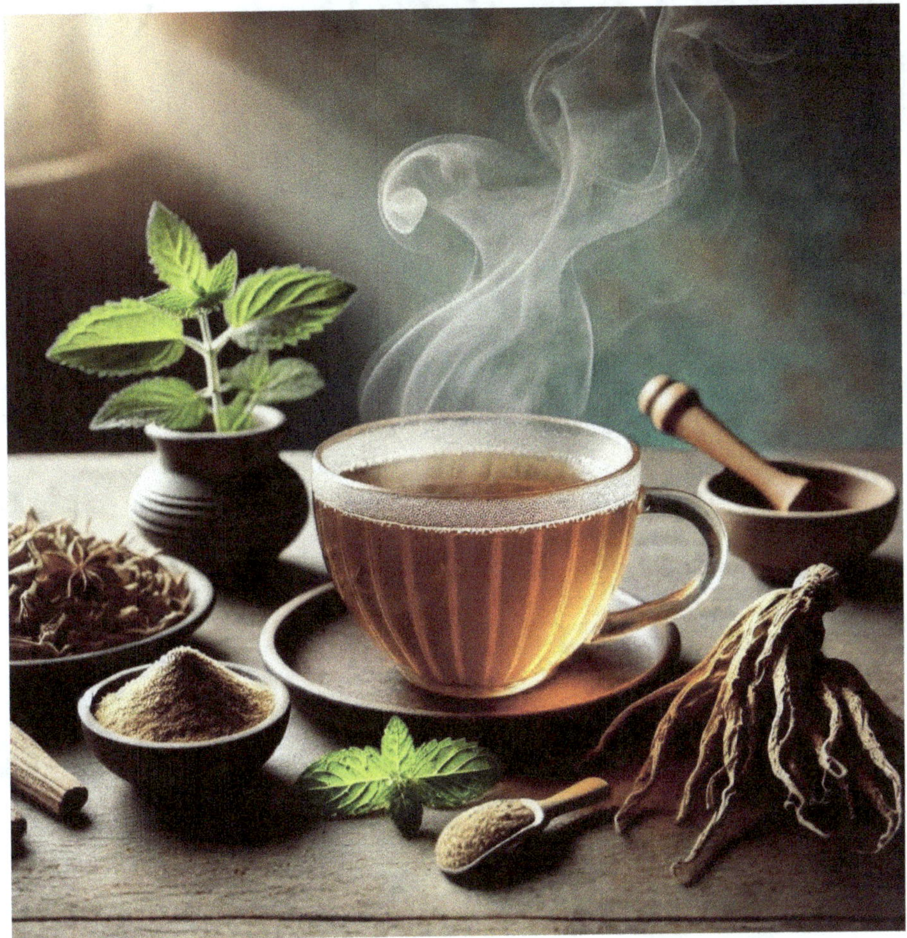

Ingredients:

- 1 teaspoon dried ashwagandha root or ½ teaspoon ashwagandha powder
- 1 cup water
- Honey or cinnamon (optional, for taste)
- A few fresh mint leaves (optional)

1. In a small saucepan, combine ashwagandha root (or powder) and water.
2. Bring to a boil over medium heat.
3. Reduce heat and simmer for 10–15 minutes.
4. Remove from heat and add mint leaves if using; let steep for an additional 5 minutes.
5. Strain the tea into a cup.
6. Add honey or a pinch of cinnamon if desired.
7. Sip slowly, embracing a moment of calm.

Usage:

- Drink one cup daily to help reduce stress and enhance energy levels.
- Ideal in the morning or early afternoon.

Caution:

- **Medical Conditions:** Consult a healthcare provider if you have autoimmune diseases or are taking thyroid medications.
- **Pregnancy and Breastfeeding:** Not recommended without professional guidance.
- **Sedative Effects:** May cause drowsiness in some individuals.

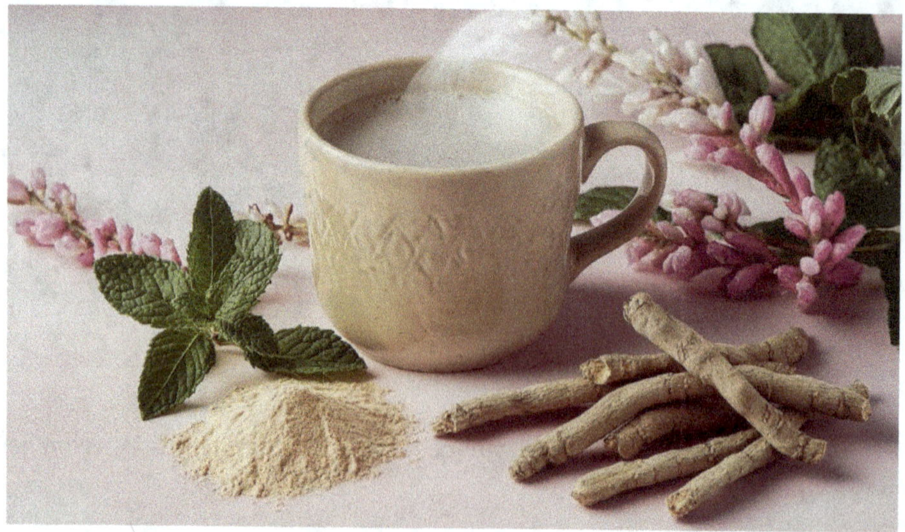

Recipe 48: Rhodiola Adaptogenic Tonic

Rhodiola rosea, native to the cold regions of Europe and Asia, has been used for centuries to fight fatigue, enhance mental performance, and improve resilience to stress. As an adaptogen, rhodiola helps balance cortisol levels, promoting sustained energy without the jitteriness associated with stimulants. This tonic is a revitalizing way to incorporate rhodiola into your wellness regimen.

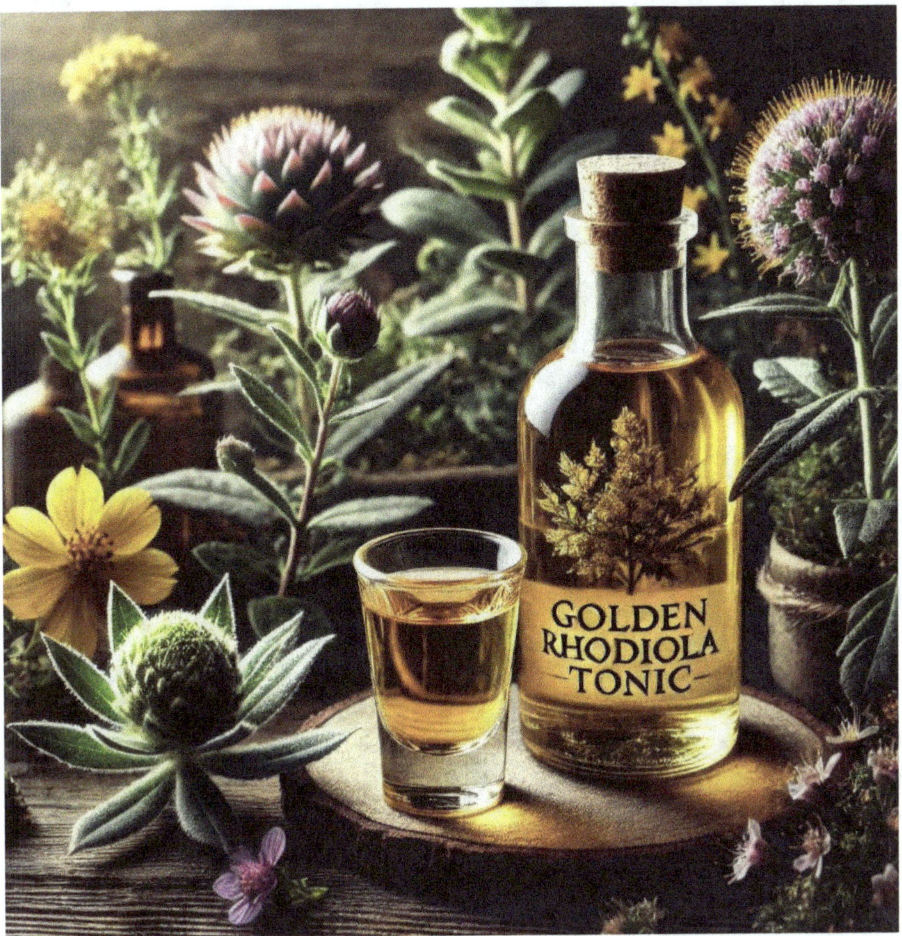

Ingredients:

- 1 tablespoon dried rhodiola root
- 2 cups water
- 1 tablespoon honey (optional)
- Juice of half a lemon (optional)

Instructions:

1. Combine dried rhodiola root and water in a saucepan.
2. Bring to a gentle boil over medium heat.
3. Reduce heat and simmer for 15–20 minutes.
4. Remove from heat and let steep until cool.
5. Strain the liquid into a glass bottle or jar.
6. Stir in honey and lemon juice if desired.
7. Store in the refrigerator for up to one week.

Usage:

- Take 1–2 ounces of the tonic once or twice daily.
- Best consumed in the morning or early afternoon to avoid interference with sleep.

Caution:

- **Medical Conditions:** Consult a healthcare provider if you have bipolar disorder or are taking antidepressants.
- **Pregnancy and Breastfeeding:** Safety not well-established; seek professional advice.
- **Side Effects:** May cause dizziness or dry mouth in some individuals.

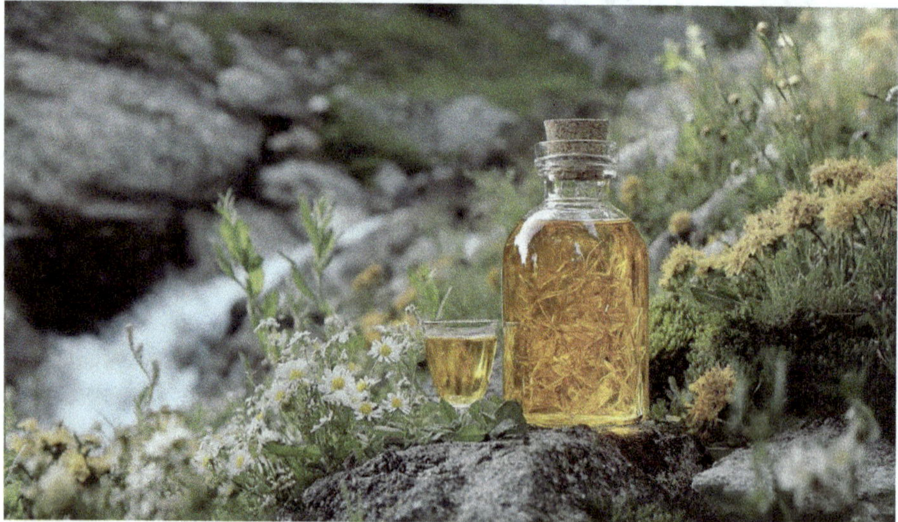

Recipe 49: Holy Basil (Tulsi) Balancing Infusion

Holy basil, or tulsi, is revered in Ayurvedic tradition as an "elixir of life" for its restorative properties. Known to reduce stress, enhance mental clarity, and support immune function, tulsi is an adaptogen that promotes overall vitality. This aromatic infusion offers a fragrant and calming experience that energizes the mind and body.

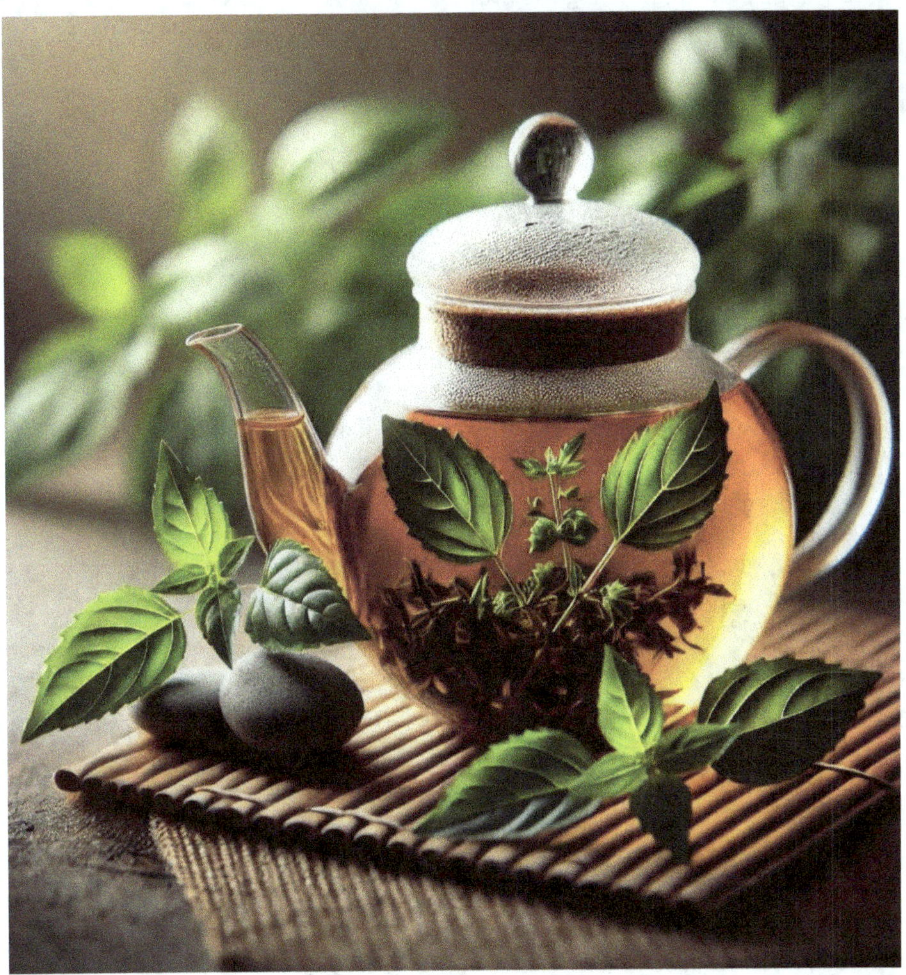

Ingredients:

- 1 tablespoon fresh holy basil leaves or 1 teaspoon dried leaves
- 1 cup boiling water
- Honey or lemon (optional)

1. Place holy basil leaves in a teapot or infuser.
2. Pour boiling water over the leaves.
3. Cover and let steep for 5–10 minutes.
4. Strain the infusion into a cup.
5. Add honey or lemon if desired.
6. Enjoy warm, inhaling the aromatic steam.

Usage:

- Drink 1–2 cups daily to promote energy, mental clarity, and stress resilience.
- Suitable for any time of day.

Caution:

- **Blood Sugar Levels:** May lower blood sugar; diabetics should monitor levels closely.
- **Pregnancy and Breastfeeding:** Generally considered safe, but consult a healthcare provider.
- **Allergies:** Check for potential sensitivity to basil or mint family plants.

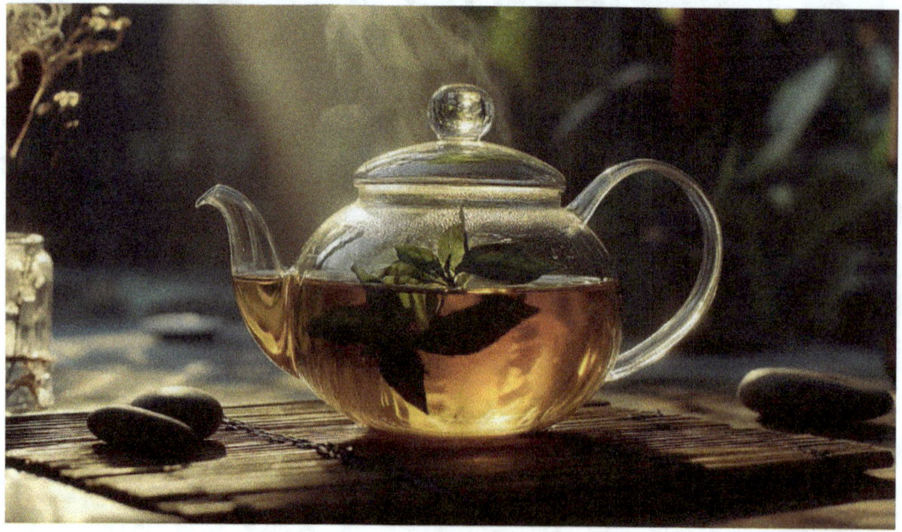

Recipe 50: Schisandra Berry Vitality Elixir

Schisandra berries, known as "wu wei zi" or "five-flavor fruit" in Traditional Chinese Medicine, are esteemed for their harmonizing effects on the body's systems. Believed to enhance energy, improve mental performance, and promote longevity, schisandra is a powerful adaptogen. This flavorful elixir combines the tartness of the berries with a hint of sweetness for a rejuvenating drink.

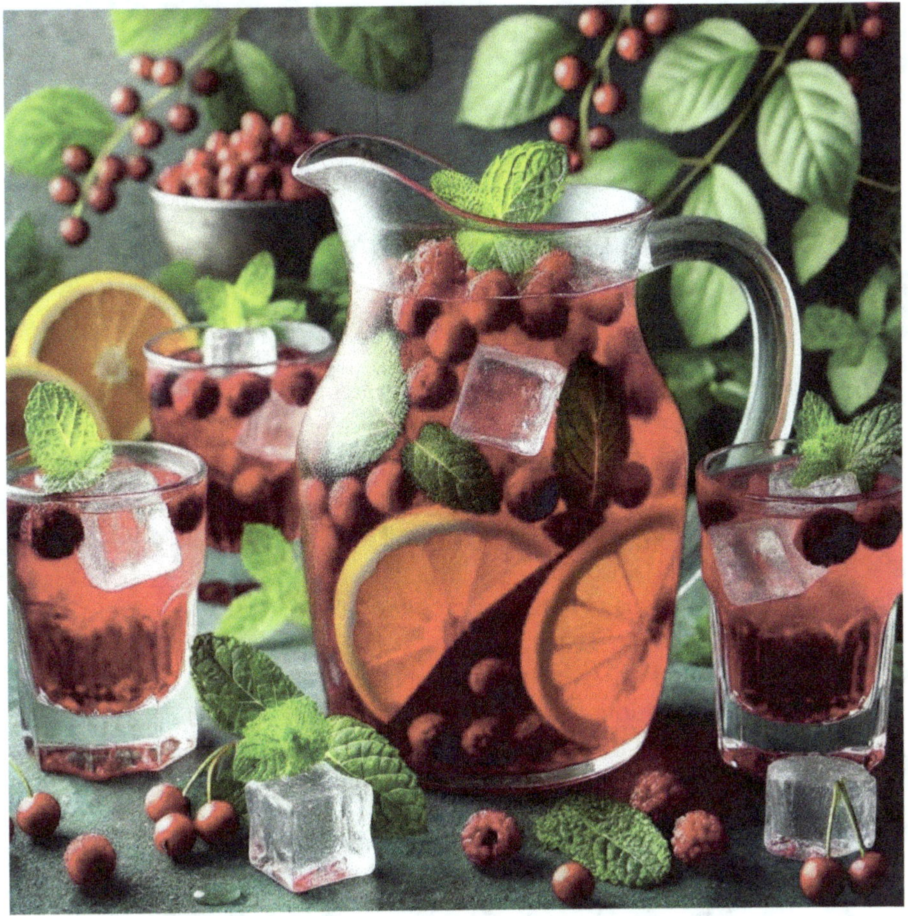

Ingredients:

- ¼ cup dried schisandra berries
- 4 cups water
- 2 tablespoons honey or agave syrup
- Juice of one orange or lemon
- Ice and fresh mint leaves for serving (optional)

Instructions:

1. Rinse the dried schisandra berries under cool water.
2. In a saucepan, combine berries and water.
3. Bring to a boil, then reduce heat and simmer for 20 minutes.
4. Remove from heat and let the mixture cool.
5. Strain the liquid into a pitcher, pressing the berries to extract all juice.
6. Stir in honey or agave syrup and citrus juice.
7. Chill in the refrigerator.
8. Serve over ice with fresh mint leaves if desired.

Usage:

- Enjoy a glass in the morning or midday to boost energy and support overall vitality.
- Can be stored refrigerated for up to three days.

Caution:

- **Medications:** Consult a healthcare provider if taking medications metabolized by the liver, as schisandra may affect liver enzymes.
- **Pregnancy and Breastfeeding:** Avoid use unless under professional supervision.
- **Allergies:** Rare, but discontinue use if any adverse reactions occur.

Note: The recipes in this chapter are designed to support energy levels and vitality through natural, herbal means. Individual responses to herbs can vary. It's important to use these remedies as part of a balanced lifestyle that includes proper nutrition, exercise, and rest. Always consult a qualified healthcare professional before starting any new herbal regimen, especially if you have underlying health conditions or are taking medications.

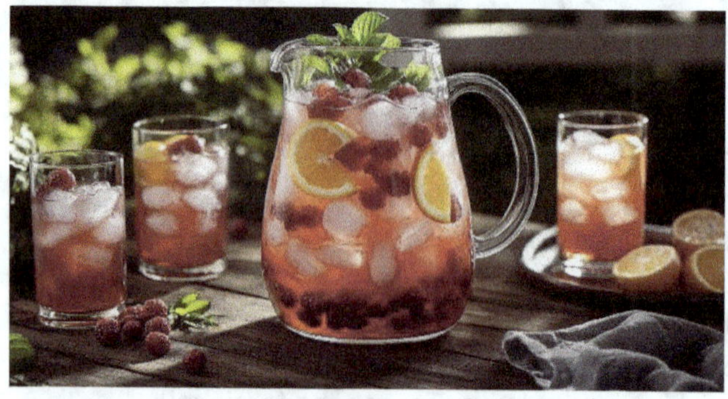

Chapter 11: Detoxification

Recipe 51: Milk Thistle Liver Support Tea

Milk thistle, with its vibrant purple flowers and distinctive milky-veined leaves, has been used for over 2,000 years as a natural remedy for liver support. Native to the Mediterranean region, this herb contains silymarin, a compound believed to promote liver health by protecting liver cells from toxins and aiding in regeneration. A gentle milk thistle tea offers a soothing way to support your body's natural cleansing processes.

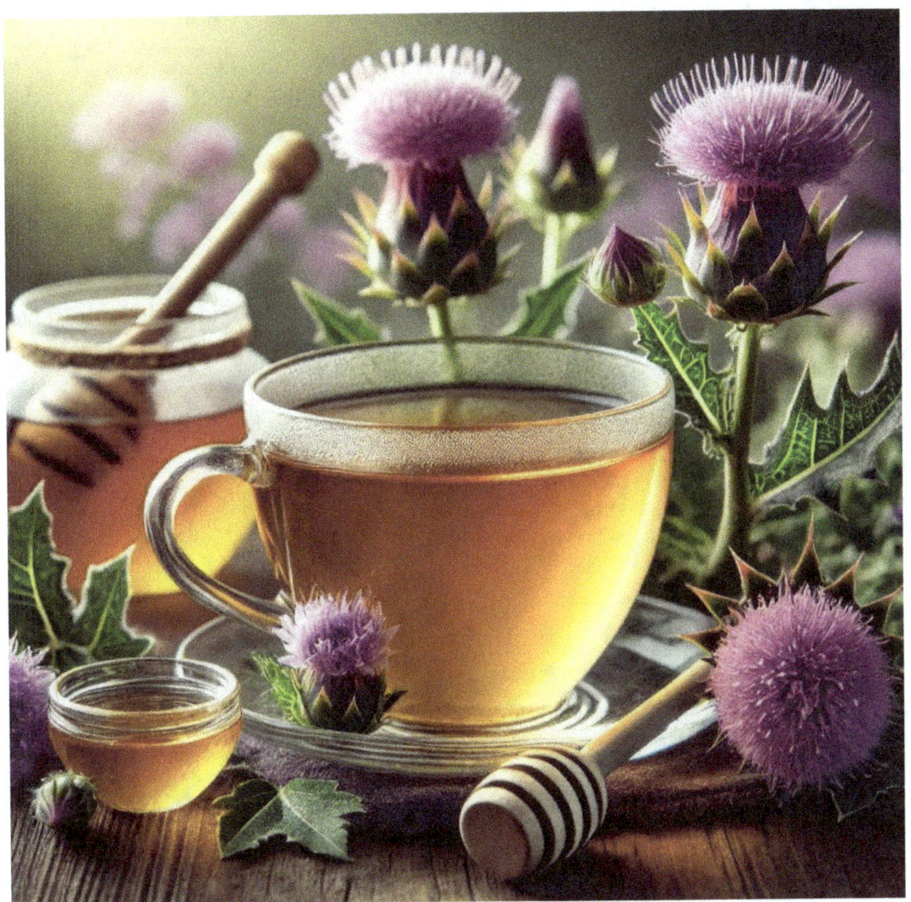

Ingredients:

- 1 tablespoon crushed milk thistle seeds
- 1 cup boiling water
- Honey or lemon (optional, for taste)

1. Place the crushed milk thistle seeds in a teapot or infuser.
2. Pour boiling water over the seeds.
3. Cover and let steep for 15–20 minutes to extract the beneficial compounds.
4. Strain the tea into a cup.
5. Add honey or lemon if desired.
6. Sip slowly, appreciating the subtle, nutty flavor.

Usage:

- Drink one cup daily to support liver health.
- Best consumed in the morning or between meals.

Caution:

- **Allergies:** Avoid if allergic to plants in the Asteraceae family (e.g., ragweed, daisies).
- **Medical Conditions:** Consult a healthcare provider if you have hormone-sensitive conditions, as milk thistle may have estrogenic effects.
- **Pregnancy and Breastfeeding:** Safety is not well-established; consult a professional before use.

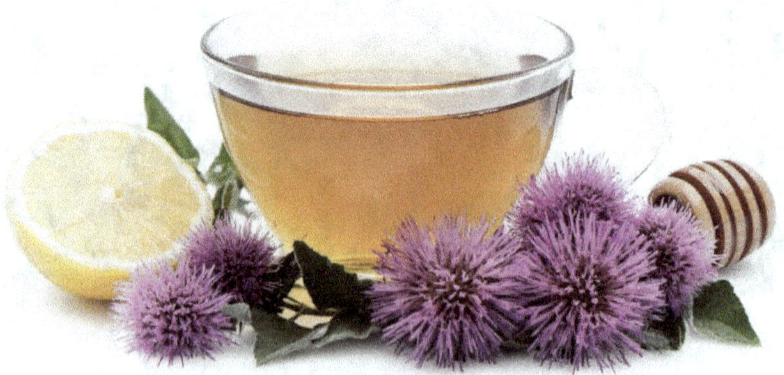

Recipe 52: Burdock Root Cleansing Decoction

Burdock root, a staple in traditional Chinese and European herbal medicine, is known for its potential to purify the blood and support the lymphatic system. Rich in antioxidants and inulin, a prebiotic fiber, burdock may aid in eliminating toxins and promoting healthy digestion. This earthy decoction harnesses the root's properties in a warm, comforting drink.

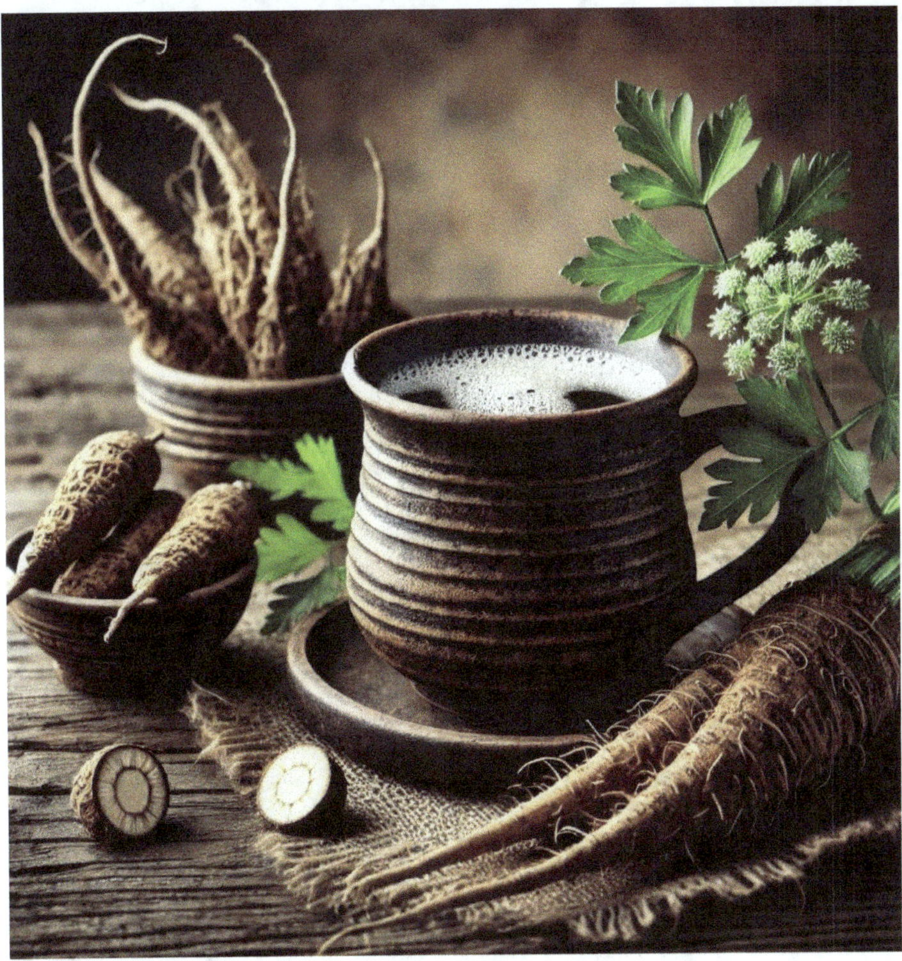

Ingredients:

- 1 tablespoon dried burdock root, sliced
- 2 cups water
- Optional: A slice of fresh ginger for added flavor

Instructions:

1. Combine burdock root (and ginger if using) with water in a saucepan.
2. Bring to a boil over medium heat.
3. Reduce heat and simmer gently for 20–30 minutes.
4. Remove from heat and let steep for an additional 10 minutes.
5. Strain the liquid into a cup.
6. Enjoy warm, optionally adding a touch of honey to sweeten.

Usage:

- Drink one cup once or twice daily for a gentle cleansing effect.
- Can be consumed over a period of one to two weeks.

Caution:

- **Allergies:** Avoid if allergic to burdock or related plants (e.g., daisies, chrysanthemums).
- **Medical Conditions:** Consult a healthcare provider if you have diabetes, as burdock may lower blood sugar levels.
- **Pregnancy and Breastfeeding:** Not recommended due to insufficient safety data.

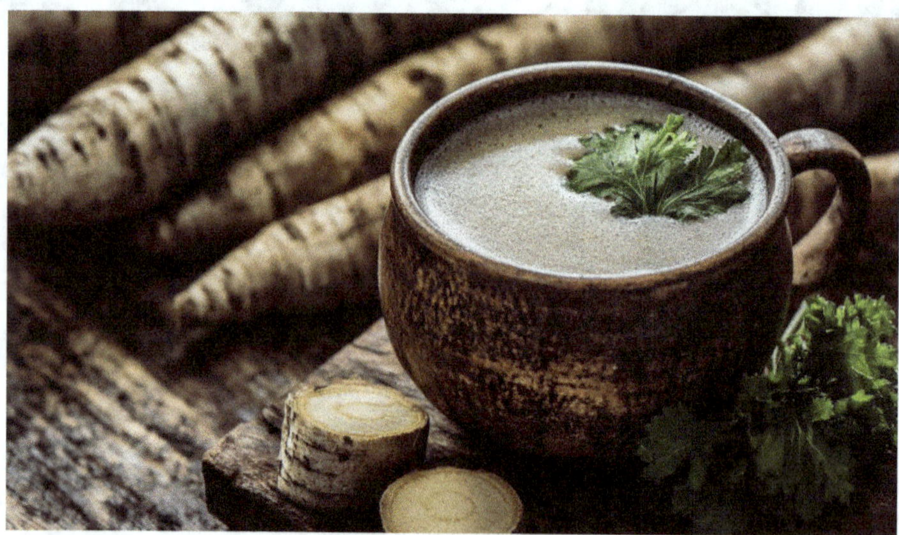

Recipe 53: Dandelion and Nettle Revitalizing Smoothie

Often dismissed as mere weeds, dandelion and nettle are powerhouses of nutrition and have been used traditionally to support the body's natural detoxification processes. Dandelion supports liver and kidney function, while nettle is rich in vitamins and minerals that nourish the body. This vibrant smoothie combines these two herbs with fresh fruits for a refreshing and revitalizing drink.

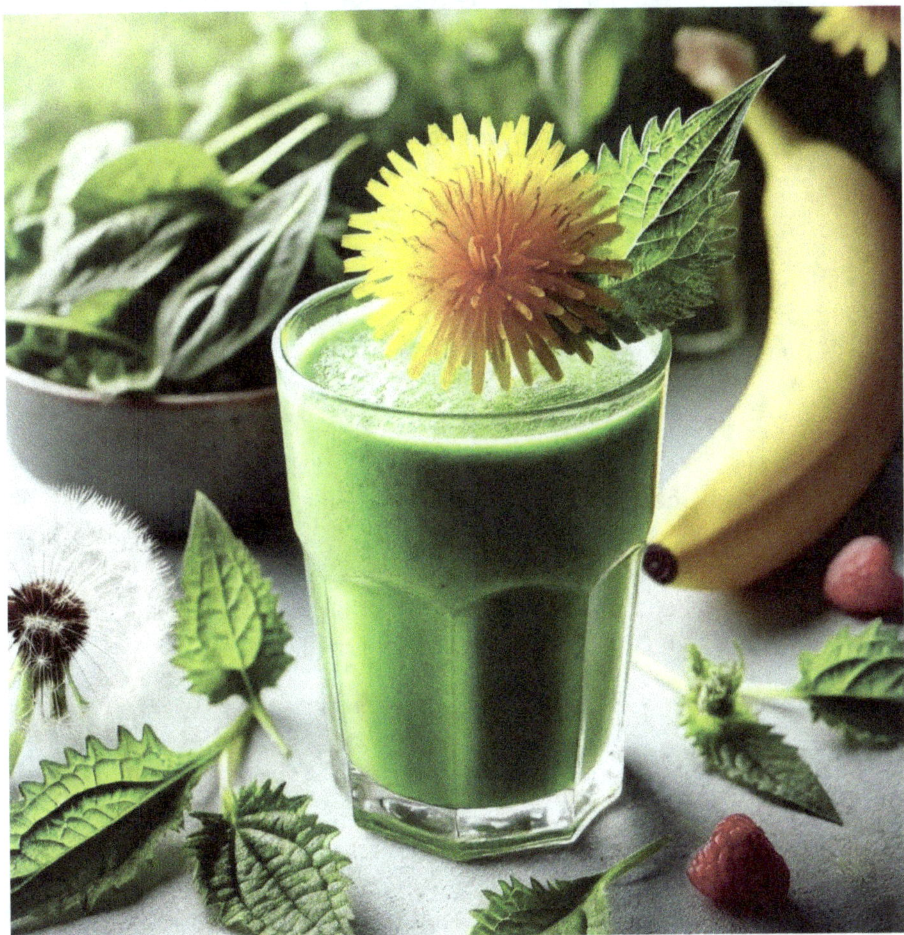

Ingredients:

- 1 handful fresh nettle leaves (using gloves to handle) or 1 teaspoon dried nettle
- 1 handful fresh dandelion greens
- 1 ripe banana

- ½ cup fresh or frozen berries (e.g., strawberries, blueberries)
- 1 cup water or coconut water
- Juice of half a lemon
- 1 teaspoon honey or maple syrup (optional, for sweetness)

Instructions:

1. If using fresh nettle, blanch the leaves in boiling water for 1 minute to neutralize the sting, then rinse with cold water.
2. Place all ingredients into a blender.
3. Blend on high until smooth and creamy.
4. Taste and adjust sweetness or acidity as desired.
5. Pour into a glass and enjoy immediately.

Usage:

- Enjoy this smoothie as a nutritious breakfast or midday snack to support overall wellness.
- Can be consumed several times a week.

Caution:

- **Allergies:** Check for potential allergies to nettle or dandelion.
- **Medical Conditions:** Consult a healthcare provider if you have kidney issues or are taking diuretics.
- **Pregnancy and Breastfeeding:** Generally considered safe in food amounts, but consult a professional for medicinal use.

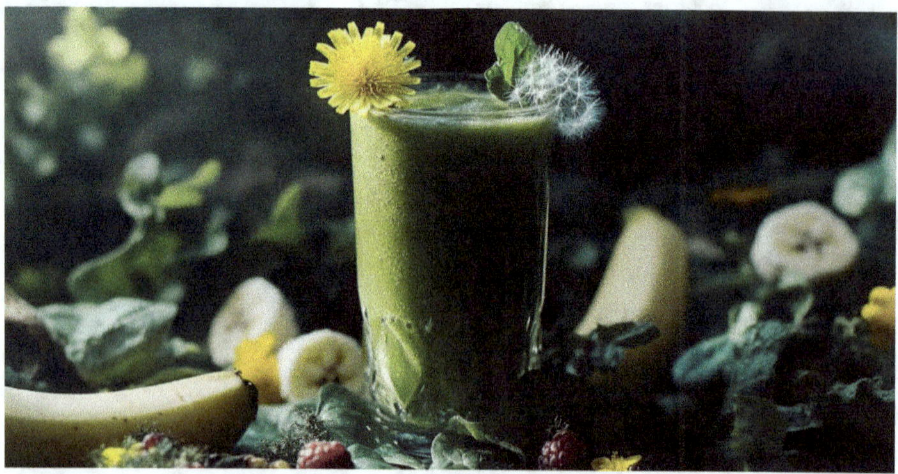

Recipe 54: Cilantro and Parsley Heavy Metal Cleanse Juice

Cilantro and parsley are more than culinary herbs; they have been studied for their potential to support the body's elimination of heavy metals. Rich in chlorophyll and antioxidants, these herbs may bind to toxins and aid in their removal. This fresh juice blends them with hydrating cucumber and apple for a crisp, detoxifying drink.

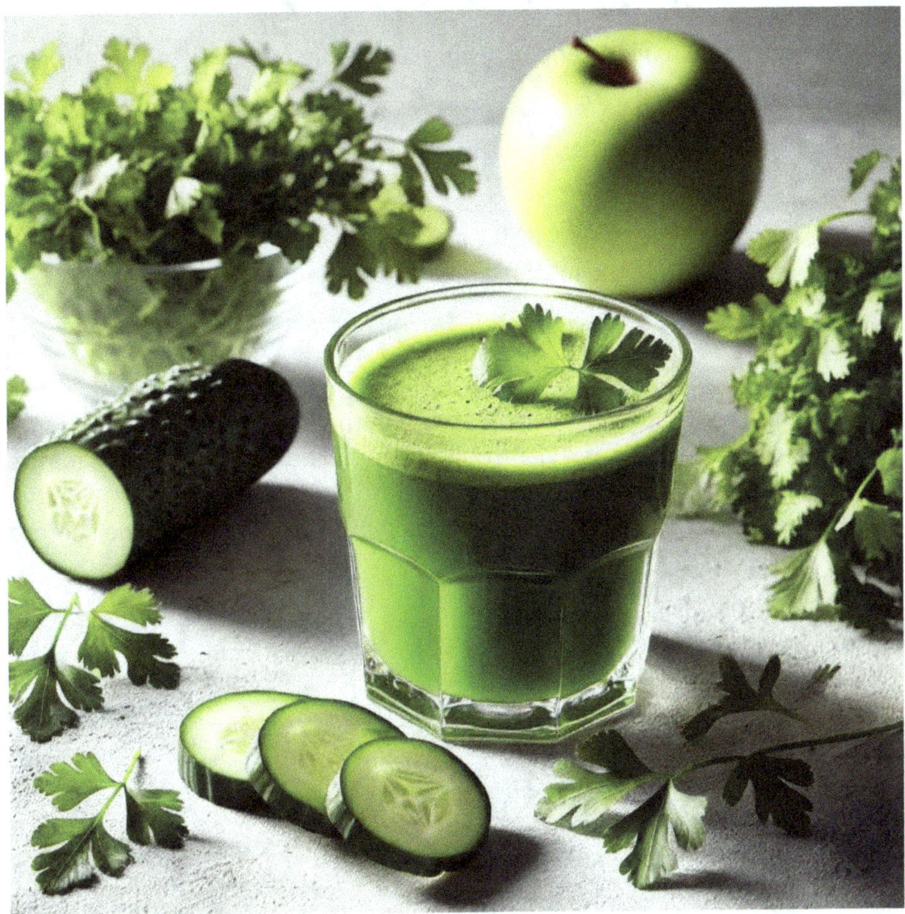

Ingredients:

- 1 large handful fresh cilantro leaves
- 1 large handful fresh parsley leaves
- 1 cucumber, peeled and chopped
- 1 green apple, cored and sliced
- Juice of one lemon
- A small piece of fresh ginger (optional, for zing)

1. Wash all fresh produce thoroughly.
2. Pass the cilantro, parsley, cucumber, apple, and ginger (if using) through a juicer.
   - Alternatively, blend all ingredients with a small amount of water in a high-speed blender until smooth, then strain through a fine mesh strainer or nut milk bag.
3. Stir in the lemon juice.
4. Pour into a glass and consume immediately to retain maximum nutrients.

Usage:

- Drink this juice once daily for a week as part of a balanced diet.
- Best enjoyed in the morning on an empty stomach.

Caution:

- **Allergies:** Ensure no allergies to any of the ingredients.
- **Medical Conditions:** Cilantro may affect blood sugar levels; diabetics should monitor accordingly.
- **Pregnancy and Breastfeeding:** Consult a healthcare provider before use.

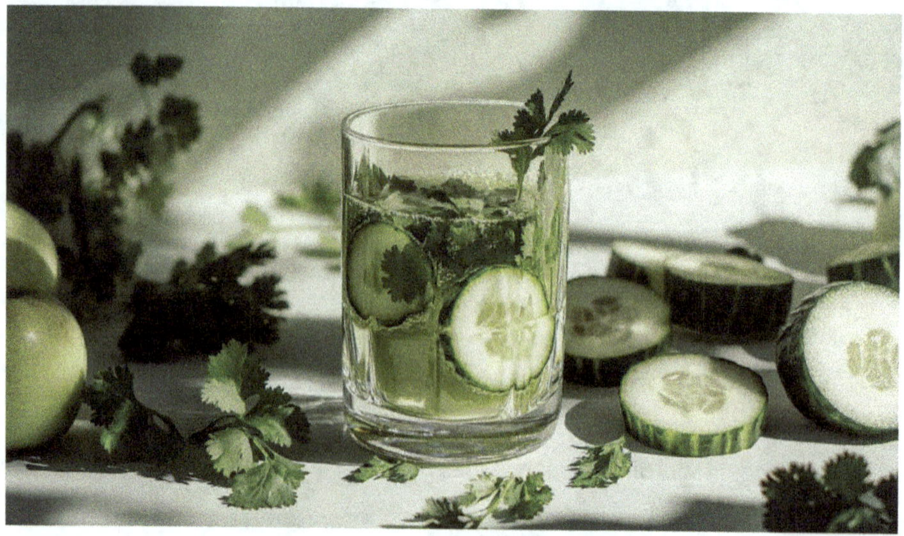

Recipe 55: Lemon and Ginger Cleansing Water

Simple yet effective, lemon and ginger water is a classic recipe to support digestion and hydration. Lemon provides vitamin C and aids in stimulating the digestive system, while ginger offers anti-inflammatory properties and soothes the gut. Sipping this infused water throughout the day can help maintain hydration and gently encourage the body's natural detox processes.

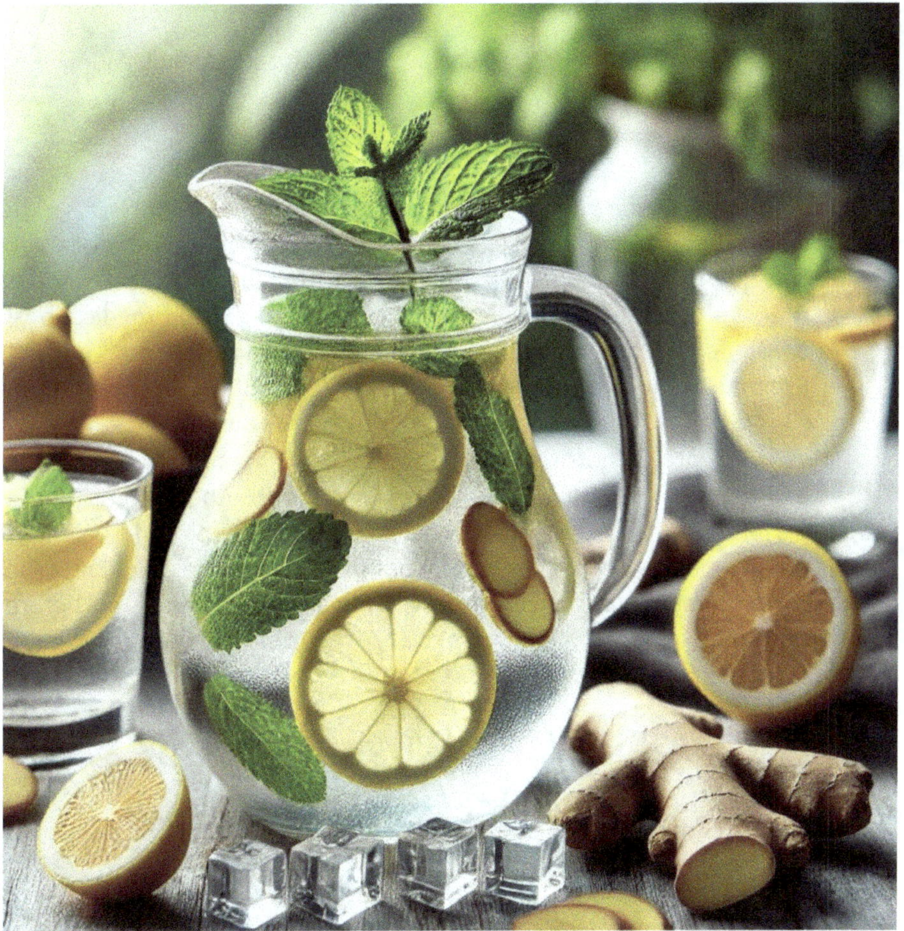

Ingredients:

- 1 lemon, thinly sliced
- 1-inch piece of fresh ginger root, peeled and sliced
- 1 pitcher (about 8 cups) of filtered water
- Optional: Fresh mint leaves or a dash of cayenne pepper

Instructions:

1. Place the lemon slices and ginger into the pitcher of water.
2. Add mint leaves or a pinch of cayenne pepper if desired.
3. Stir gently and refrigerate for at least 1 hour to allow flavors to infuse.
4. Serve cold, pouring into individual glasses over ice if preferred.

Usage:

- Drink throughout the day to stay hydrated and support digestion.
- Can be made fresh daily.

Caution:

- **Dental Health:** Prolonged exposure to lemon can affect tooth enamel; consider using a straw and rinsing mouth after consumption.
- **Medical Conditions:** Ginger may interact with certain medications; consult a healthcare provider if taking blood thinners.
- **Pregnancy and Breastfeeding:** Generally safe, but moderation is key.

Note: The concept of "detoxification" in the body primarily refers to the natural processes carried out by the liver, kidneys, and other organs. These recipes are intended to support overall health and should be part of a balanced diet and healthy lifestyle. They are not meant to replace professional medical advice or treatment. Always consult a qualified healthcare professional before starting any new health regimen, especially if you have underlying health conditions or are taking medications.

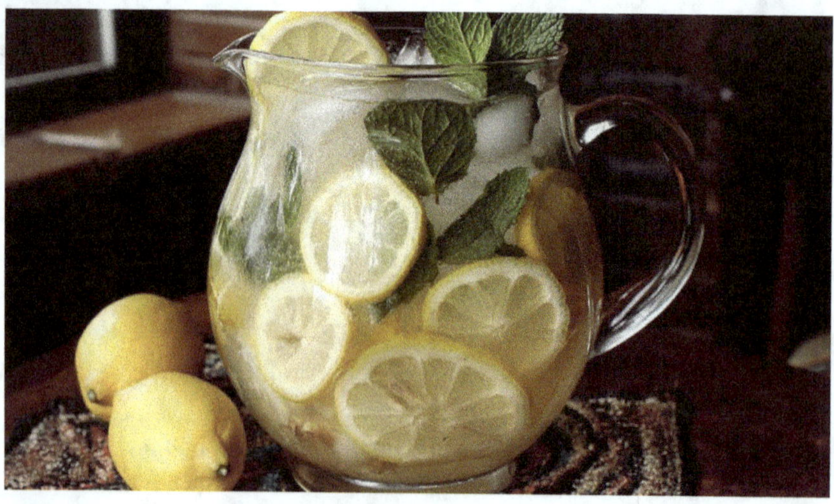

Recipe 56: Rosemary Memory Enhancement Tea

Rosemary, an aromatic herb native to the Mediterranean region, has been associated with memory and cognitive function since ancient times. Scholars in Greece and Rome are said to have worn rosemary garlands during exams to enhance memory. Modern research suggests that compounds in rosemary may support neurotransmitter activity and improve circulation to the brain. This invigorating tea offers a fragrant way to potentially boost memory and focus.

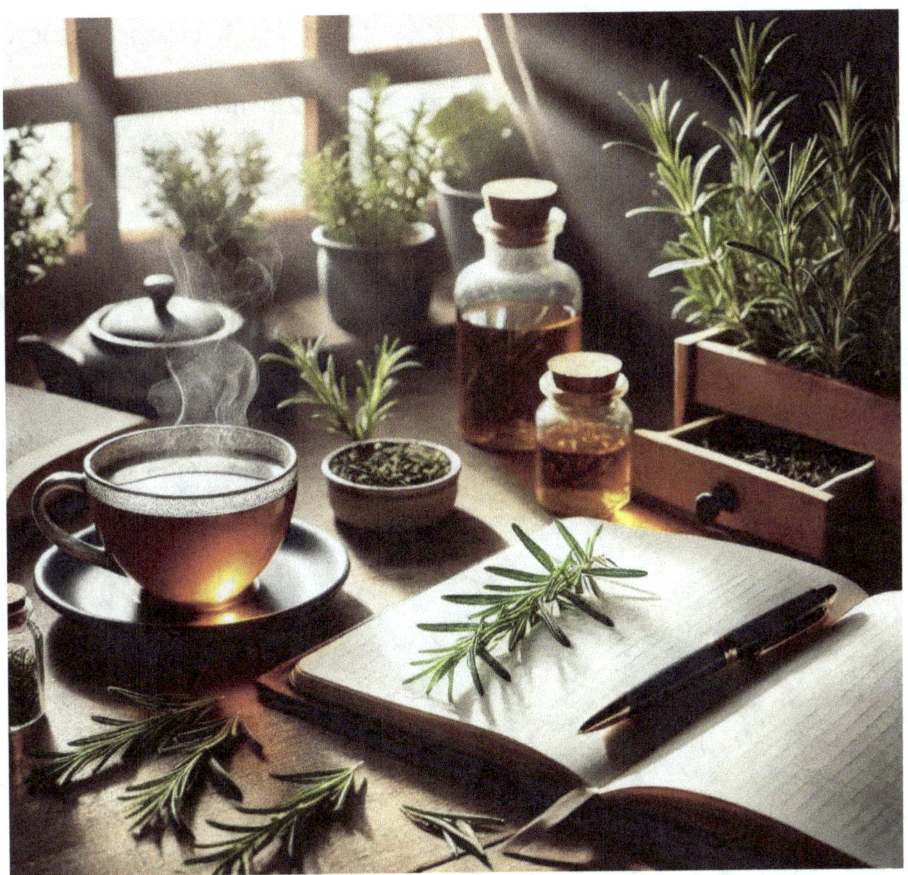

Ingredients:

- 1 teaspoon fresh rosemary leaves or ½ teaspoon dried rosemary
- 1 cup boiling water
- Honey or lemon (optional, for taste)

Instructions:

1. Rinse fresh rosemary leaves under cool water.
2. Place the rosemary in a teapot or infuser.
3. Pour boiling water over the herb.
4. Cover and let steep for 5–10 minutes to extract the aromatic oils.
5. Strain the tea into a cup.
6. Add honey or lemon if desired.
7. Sip slowly, inhaling the uplifting aroma.

Usage:

- Drink one cup in the morning or early afternoon to support memory and cognitive function.
- Ideal before study sessions or tasks requiring mental focus.

Caution:

- **Pregnancy:** Rosemary is generally safe in culinary amounts but consult a healthcare provider before using medicinal doses during pregnancy.
- **Medical Conditions:** Avoid excessive use if you have high blood pressure or epilepsy.
- **Allergies:** Check for potential sensitivity to rosemary or other members of the Lamiaceae family.

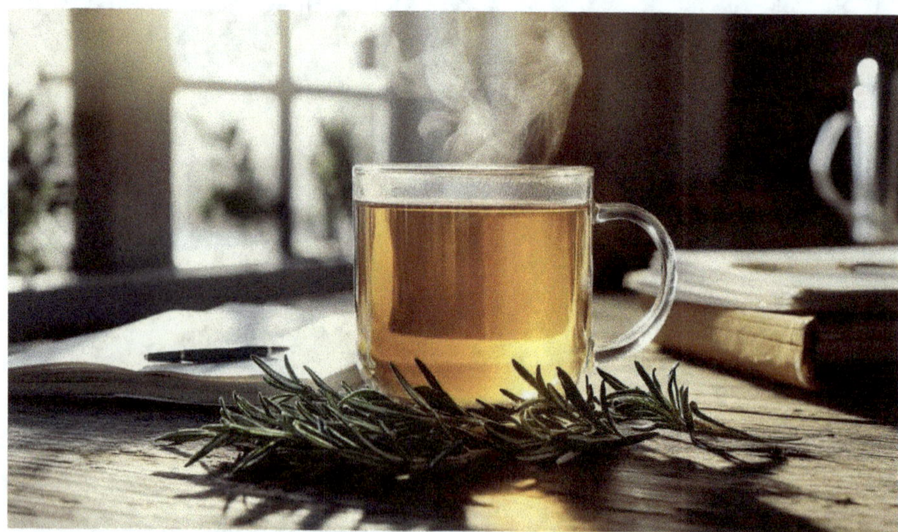

Recipe 57: Bacopa Monnieri Brain Tonic

Bacopa monnieri, also known as Brahmi, is a revered herb in Ayurvedic medicine, traditionally used to enhance learning, memory, and concentration. Native to wetlands in India and other parts of Asia, Bacopa is believed to support cognitive function by promoting neuron communication and providing antioxidant protection. This brain tonic harnesses the power of Bacopa in a simple, consumable form.

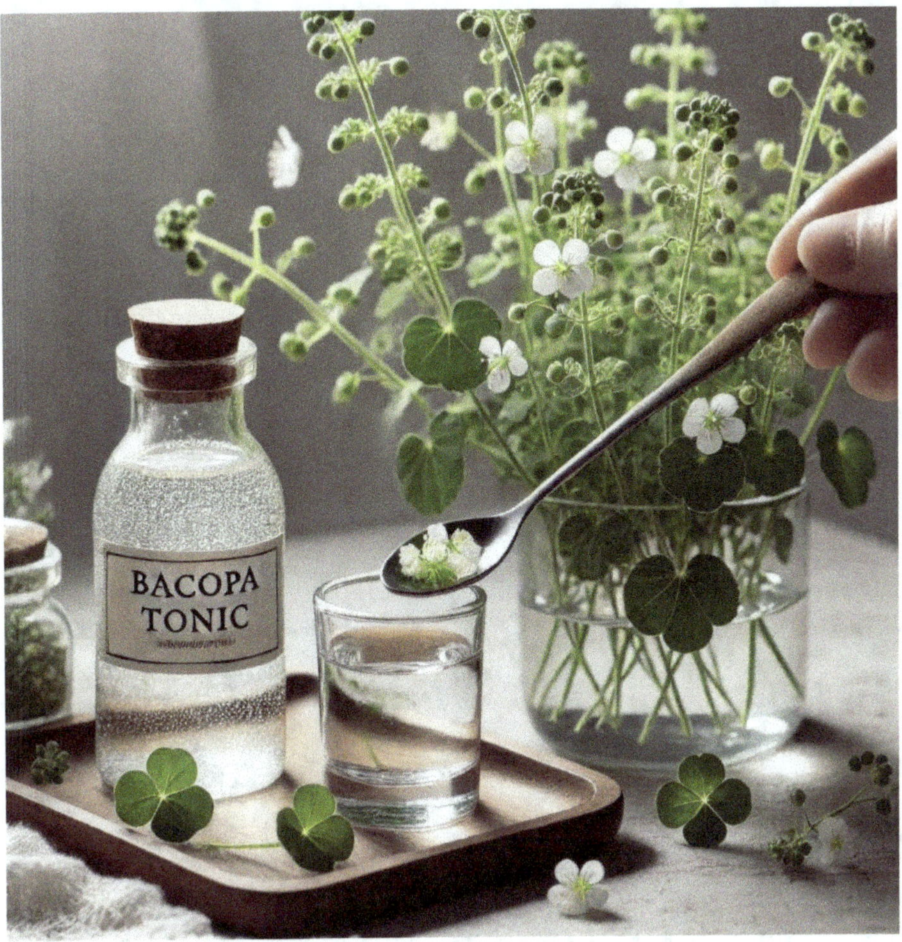

Ingredients:

- 2 teaspoons dried Bacopa monnieri leaves
- 2 cups water
- Honey or a pinch of cardamom (optional, for flavor)

1. Combine dried Bacopa leaves and water in a saucepan.
2. Bring to a gentle boil over medium heat.
3. Reduce heat and simmer for 15–20 minutes until the liquid reduces by half.
4. Remove from heat and let it cool.
5. Strain the liquid into a glass bottle or jar.
6. Add honey or cardamom if desired to improve taste.
7. Store in the refrigerator for up to one week.

Usage:

- Take 1–2 tablespoons of the tonic once or twice daily.
- Consistent use over several weeks may yield the best results for cognitive support.

Caution:

- **Medical Conditions:** Consult a healthcare provider if you have thyroid disorders or are taking medications that affect the gastrointestinal tract.
- **Side Effects:** May cause mild digestive discomfort in some individuals.
- **Pregnancy and Breastfeeding:** Safety not well-established; consult a professional before use.

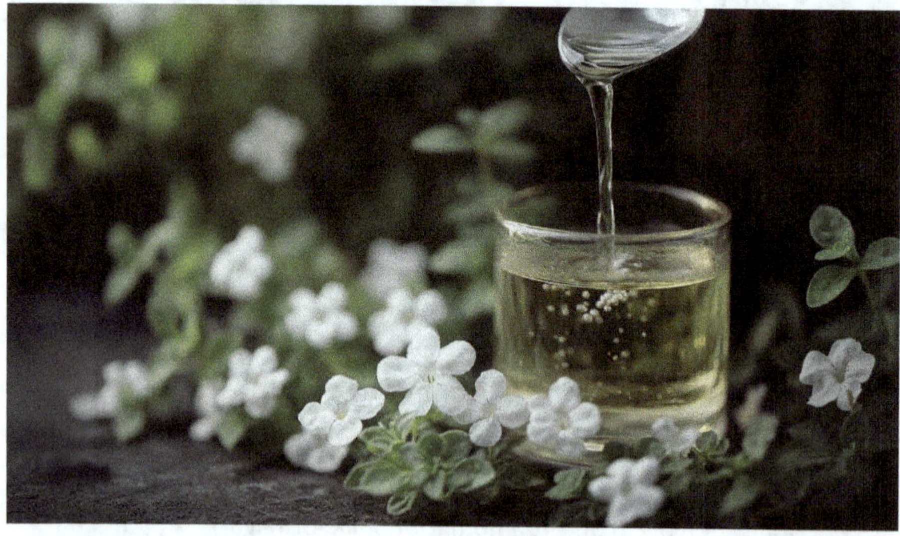

Recipe 58: Gotu Kola Concentration Aid Infusion

Gotu Kola, known as the "herb of longevity," has been a cornerstone in traditional Chinese and Ayurvedic medicine for its potential to enhance cognitive function and support nervous system health. This herb is believed to promote mental clarity, reduce anxiety, and improve circulation. An infusion of Gotu Kola offers a gentle means to potentially enhance concentration and focus.

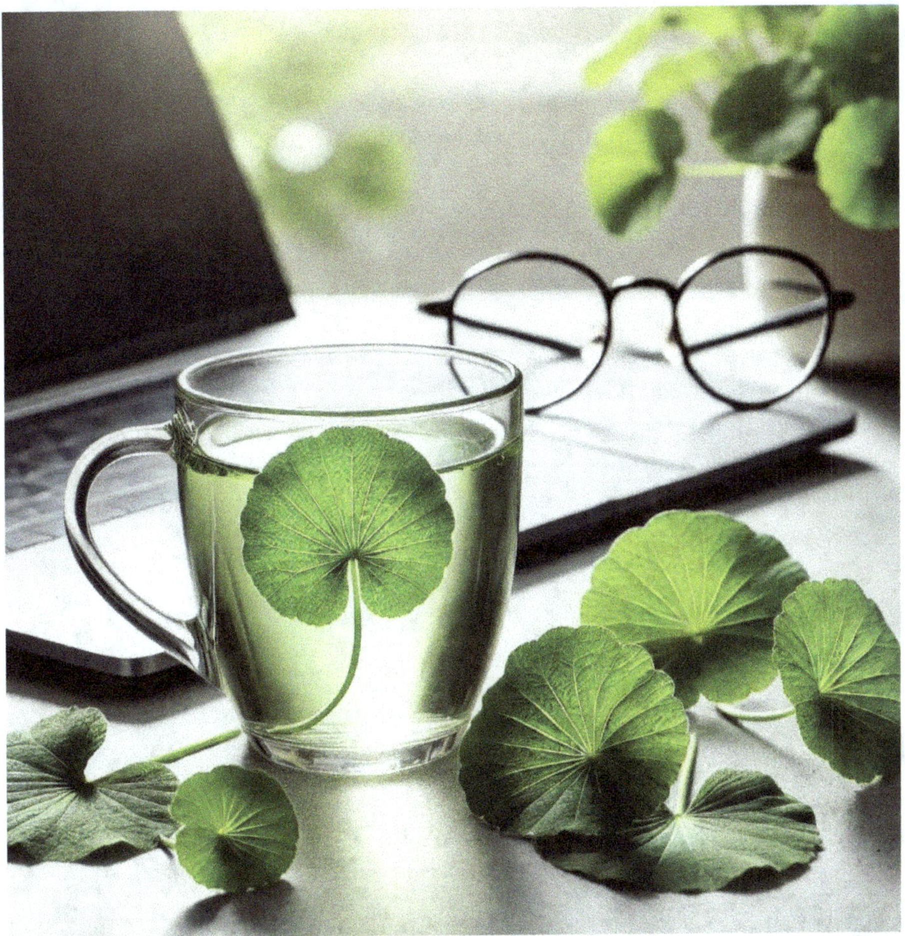

Ingredients:

- 1 teaspoon dried Gotu Kola leaves or 1 tablespoon fresh leaves
- 1 cup boiling water
- Honey or mint leaves (optional, for flavor)

Instructions:

1. Rinse fresh Gotu Kola leaves if using.
2. Place the leaves in a teapot or infuser.
3. Pour boiling water over the herb.
4. Cover and let steep for 5–10 minutes.
5. Strain the infusion into a cup.
6. Add honey or a few mint leaves if desired.
7. Enjoy warm.

Usage:

- Drink one cup up to twice daily to support concentration and mental clarity.
- Suitable for morning or early afternoon consumption.

Caution:

- **Medical Conditions:** May affect liver enzymes; consult a healthcare provider if you have liver issues.
- **Sedative Effects:** Can cause drowsiness in some individuals; avoid driving or operating heavy machinery if affected.
- **Pregnancy and Breastfeeding:** Not recommended without professional guidance.

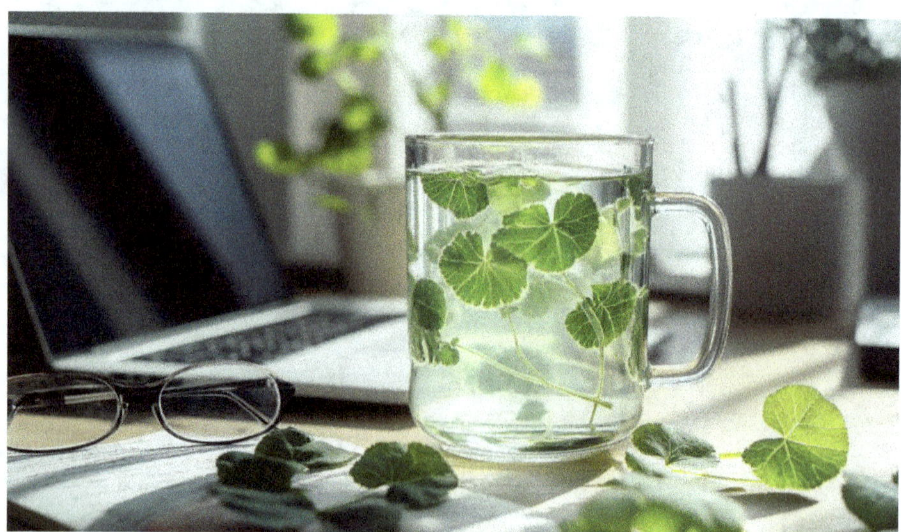

Recipe 59: Sage Cognitive Booster Tea

Sage, with its silvery leaves and earthy aroma, has a rich history of medicinal use, particularly in enhancing memory and cognitive performance. Ancient Greeks and Romans esteemed sage for its brain-boosting properties. Modern studies suggest that sage may inhibit the breakdown of acetylcholine, a neurotransmitter important for memory. This aromatic tea offers a simple way to tap into sage's potential benefits.

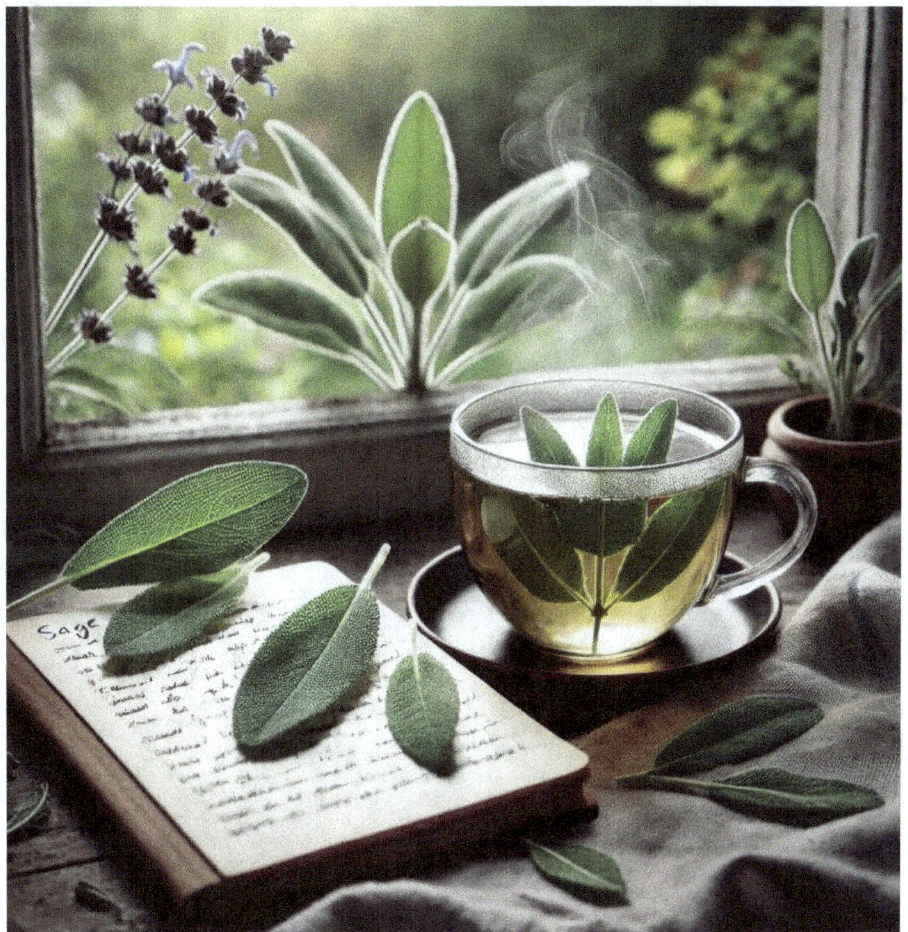

Ingredients:

- 1 teaspoon fresh sage leaves or ½ teaspoon dried sage
- 1 cup boiling water
- Lemon and honey (optional, for taste)

1. Rinse fresh sage leaves under cool water.
2. Place the sage in a teapot or infuser.
3. Pour boiling water over the herb.
4. Cover and let steep for 5–10 minutes.
5. Strain the tea into a cup.
6. Add lemon and honey if desired.
7. Sip slowly, enjoying the herbal aroma.

Usage:

- Drink one cup daily to potentially enhance cognitive function and memory.
- Ideal during study sessions or periods requiring heightened mental activity.

Caution:

- **Medical Conditions:** Avoid excessive use if you have high blood pressure or epilepsy.
- **Pregnancy and Breastfeeding:** Limit consumption, as high amounts may stimulate uterine contractions.
- **Allergies:** Ensure no sensitivity to sage or related herbs.

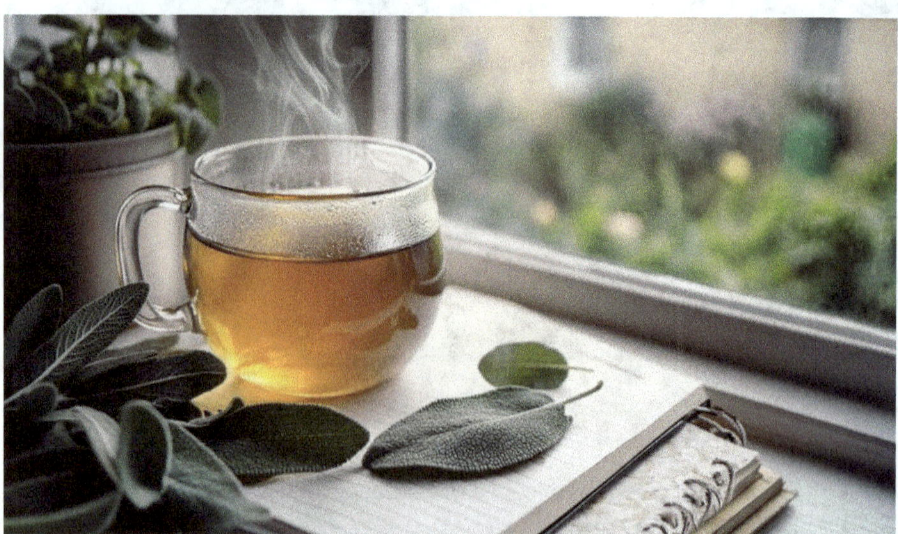

Recipe 60: Lemon Balm Focus Enhancing Elixir

Lemon balm, a lemon-scented herb from the mint family, has been used since the Middle Ages to reduce stress and anxiety, promote sleep, and improve appetite. Recent research also indicates potential cognitive benefits, such as enhancing alertness and improving mood. This refreshing elixir combines lemon balm with citrus flavors for a delightful beverage that may support focus and mental clarity.

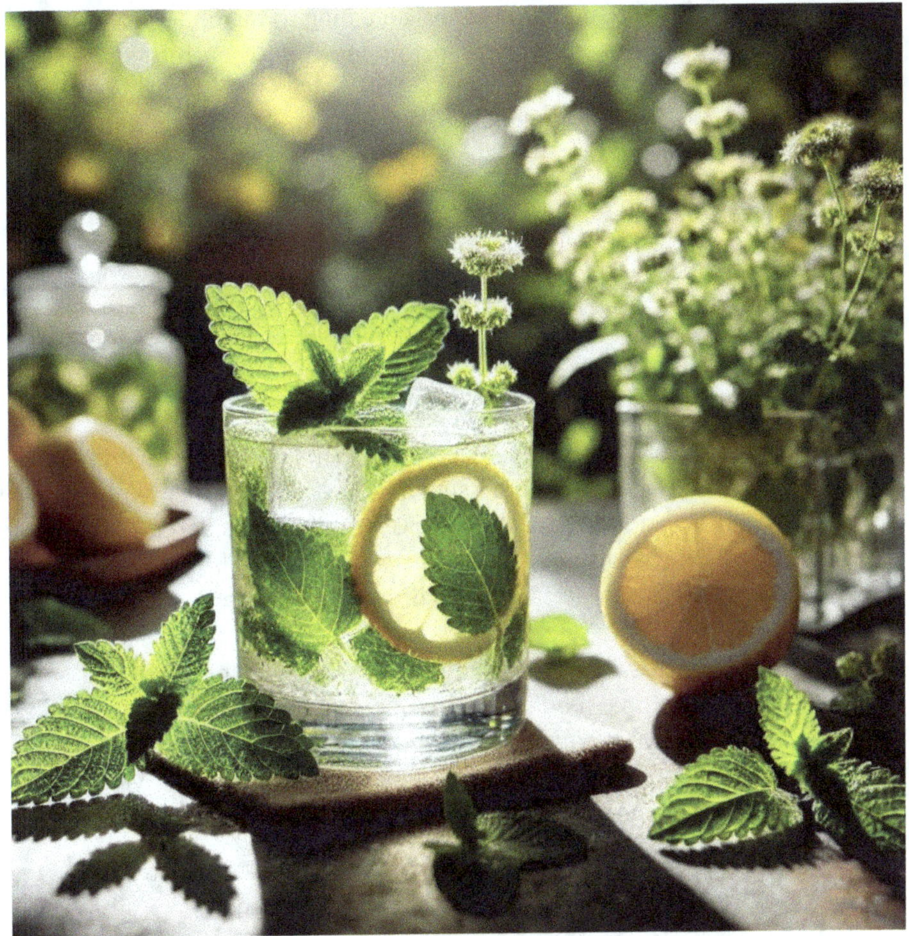

Ingredients:

- 1 cup fresh lemon balm leaves (or 2 tablespoons dried)
- 4 cups water
- Juice of one lemon
- 1–2 tablespoons honey or agave syrup

- Ice cubes
- Lemon slices and fresh mint (optional, for garnish)

Instructions:

1. In a saucepan, bring water to a boil.
2. Remove from heat and add lemon balm leaves.
3. Cover and steep for 15 minutes.
4. Strain the infusion into a pitcher.
5. Stir in lemon juice and sweetener, adjusting to taste.
6. Allow the elixir to cool to room temperature, then refrigerate until chilled.
7. Serve over ice, garnished with lemon slices and fresh mint if desired.

Usage:

- Enjoy a glass during the day to support focus and uplift the spirits.
- Suitable as a refreshing beverage during work or study breaks.

Caution:

- **Thyroid Conditions:** May affect thyroid function; consult a healthcare provider if you have thyroid issues.
- **Pregnancy and Breastfeeding:** Generally considered safe, but moderation is advised.
- **Sedative Effects:** May cause mild drowsiness in some individuals.

Note: These recipes are intended to support general wellness and are not a substitute for professional medical advice or treatment. Individual responses to herbs can vary. Always consult a qualified healthcare professional before starting any new herbal regimen, especially if you have underlying health conditions, are taking medications, or are pregnant or breastfeeding.

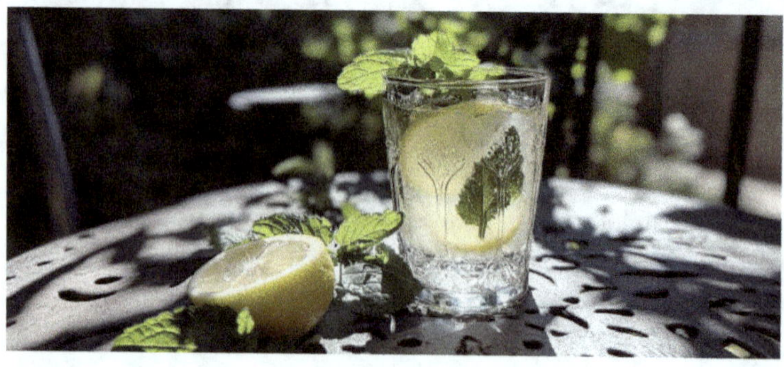

Recipe 61: Cinnamon and Clove Blood Sugar Balancing Tea

Cinnamon and clove, two aromatic spices commonly found in kitchens around the world, have been valued for their medicinal properties for centuries. Cinnamon is known for its potential to support healthy blood sugar levels by enhancing insulin sensitivity, while clove contains eugenol, which may aid in regulating glucose metabolism. This warm, spicy tea combines these two powerful spices into a delightful beverage that can be enjoyed as part of a balanced diet.

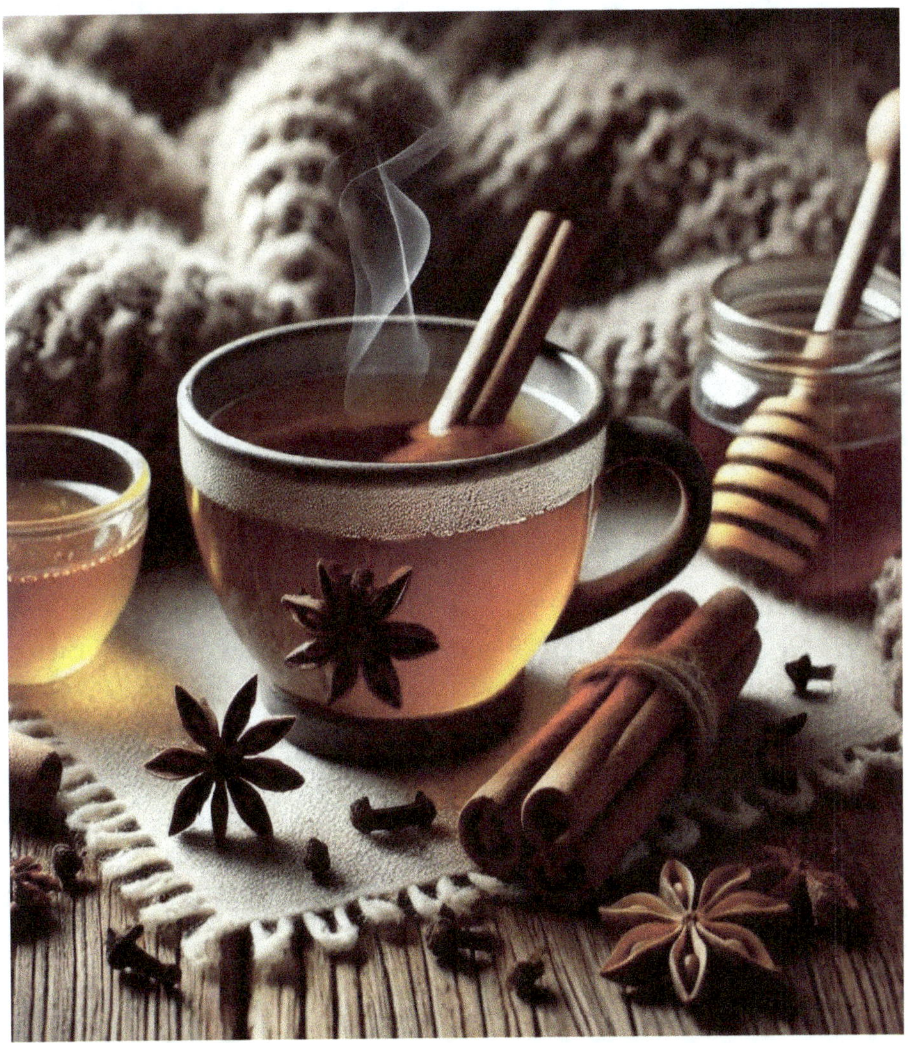

Ingredients:

- 1 cinnamon stick or 1 teaspoon ground cinnamon
- 4–5 whole cloves
- 1 cup boiling water
- Honey or stevia (optional, for sweetness)
- Lemon slice (optional, for flavor)

Instructions:

1. Place the cinnamon stick (or ground cinnamon) and whole cloves in a teapot or heatproof mug.
2. Pour boiling water over the spices.
3. Cover and let steep for 10–15 minutes to extract the full flavor and beneficial compounds.
4. Strain the tea into a cup, removing the cinnamon stick and cloves.
5. Add honey or stevia if desired for sweetness.
6. Garnish with a lemon slice if you like a hint of citrus.
7. Enjoy warm.

Usage:

- Drink one cup after meals, up to two times daily, to support healthy blood sugar levels.
- Consistent use as part of a balanced diet may offer the best results.

Caution:

- **Medical Conditions:** If you have diabetes or are taking medications that affect blood sugar, monitor your levels closely and consult a healthcare provider before use.
- **Pregnancy and Breastfeeding:** Cinnamon and clove are generally safe in culinary amounts, but high doses should be avoided; consult a professional before use.
- **Allergies:** Ensure you are not allergic to any of the ingredients.

Recipe 62: Fenugreek Seed Metabolism Boosting Infusion

Fenugreek seeds, with their slightly bitter taste and maple syrup aroma, have been used traditionally to support metabolic health and digestion. Rich in soluble fiber and compounds like trigonelline, fenugreek may help regulate blood sugar levels and improve insulin function. This simple infusion harnesses the seeds' benefits in an easy-to-consume form.

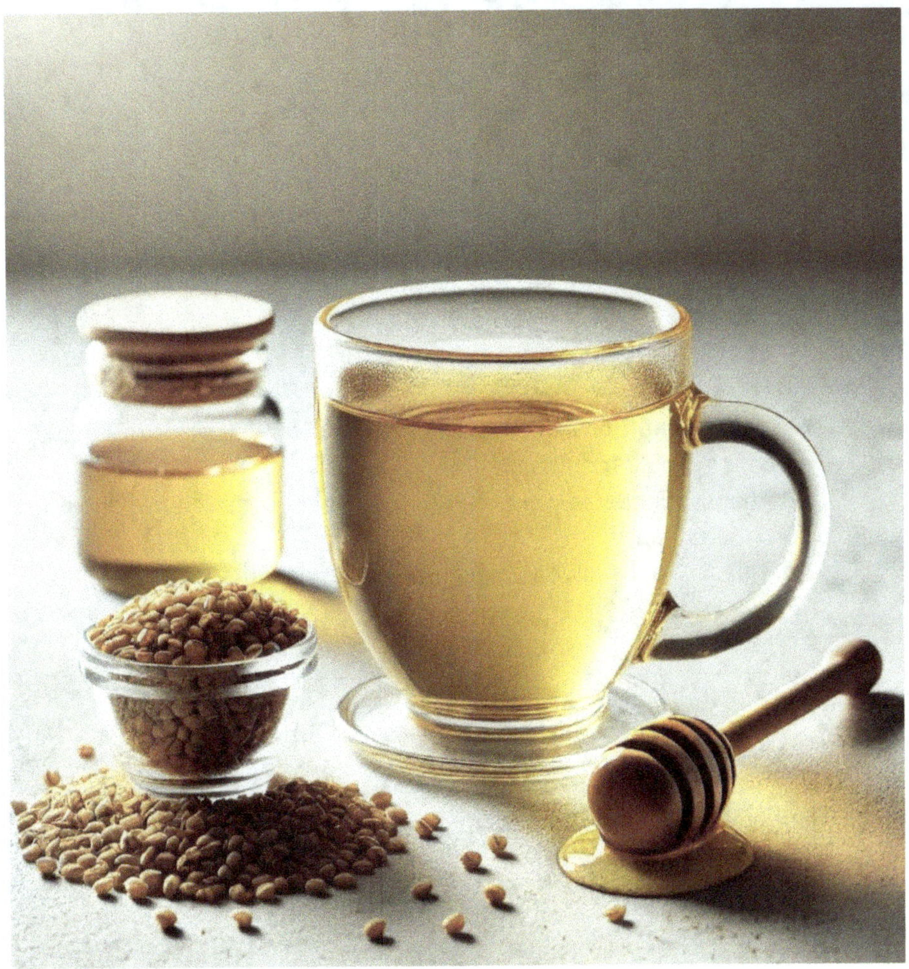

Ingredients:

- 1 teaspoon fenugreek seeds
- 1 cup boiling water
- Honey or lemon (optional, for taste)

1. Lightly crush the fenugreek seeds using a mortar and pestle to release their oils.
2. Place the crushed seeds in a teapot or infuser.
3. Pour boiling water over the seeds.
4. Cover and let steep for 15 minutes.
5. Strain the infusion into a cup.
6. Add honey or lemon if desired to enhance flavor.
7. Drink warm.

Usage:

- Consume one cup in the morning on an empty stomach to support metabolism.
- Can be taken daily as part of a balanced diet.

Caution:

- **Medical Conditions:** Fenugreek may lower blood sugar levels; diabetics should monitor their levels closely.
- **Pregnancy:** Fenugreek may stimulate uterine contractions; avoid use during pregnancy.
- **Allergies:** Avoid if allergic to legumes (e.g., peanuts, chickpeas).

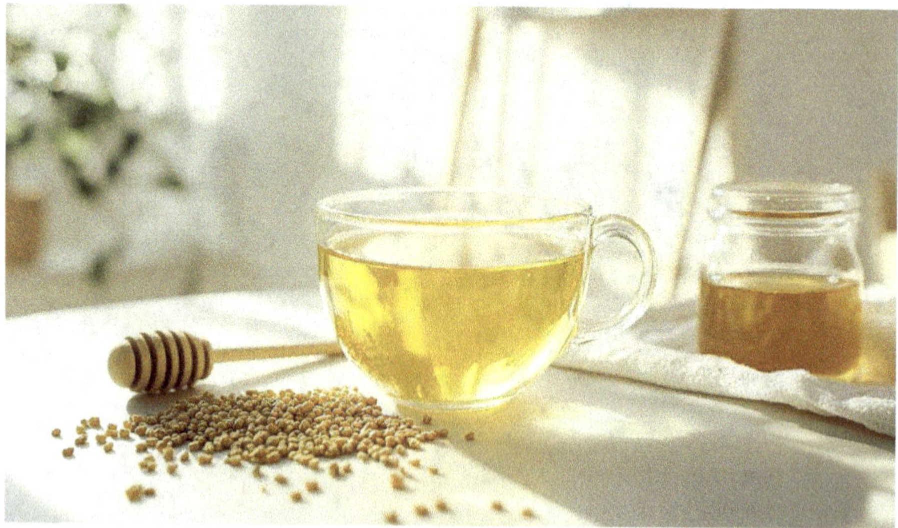

Green tea, renowned for its high antioxidant content, particularly catechins like EGCG (epigallocatechin gallate), has been associated with numerous health benefits. Regular consumption may support metabolism, promote fat oxidation, and contribute to overall wellness. This refreshing drink can be enjoyed hot or cold, making it a versatile addition to your daily routine.

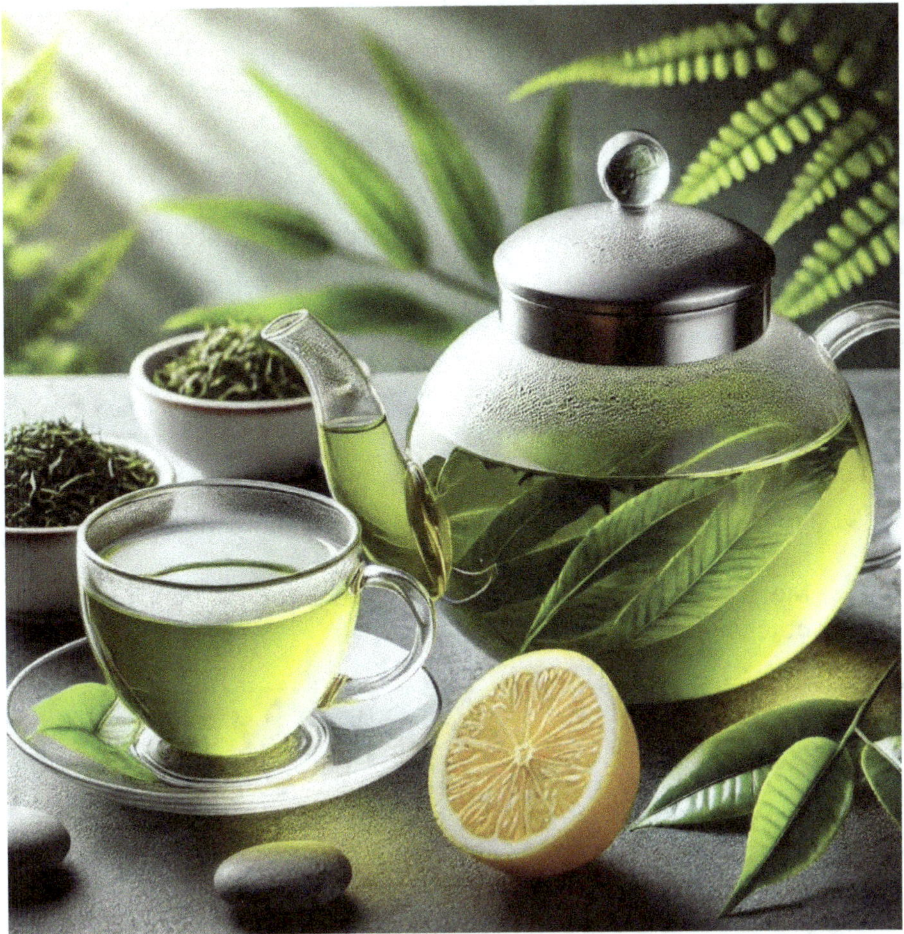

Ingredients:

- 1 teaspoon high-quality green tea leaves or 1 green tea bag
- 1 cup water (heated to about 175°F or 80°C, not boiling)
- Honey or stevia (optional)
- Lemon wedge or fresh mint (optional, for flavor)

1. Heat water to the appropriate temperature; avoid boiling to prevent bitterness.
2. Place green tea leaves or the tea bag in a teapot or cup.
3. Pour hot water over the tea.
4. Allow to steep for 2–3 minutes for optimal flavor and benefits.
5. Remove the tea leaves or bag.
6. Add sweetener if desired.
7. Garnish with a lemon wedge or mint leaves if you prefer.
8. Enjoy hot, or let it cool and serve over ice for a refreshing iced tea.

Usage:

- Drink one to three cups daily to support metabolic health and provide antioxidant benefits.
- Ideal times are in the morning and early afternoon.

Caution:

- **Caffeine Content:** Green tea contains caffeine; limit intake if sensitive or avoid consuming late in the day to prevent sleep disturbances.
- **Iron Absorption:** May inhibit iron absorption; consider consuming between meals if you have anemia.
- **Medications:** Consult a healthcare provider if taking blood thinners or other medications.

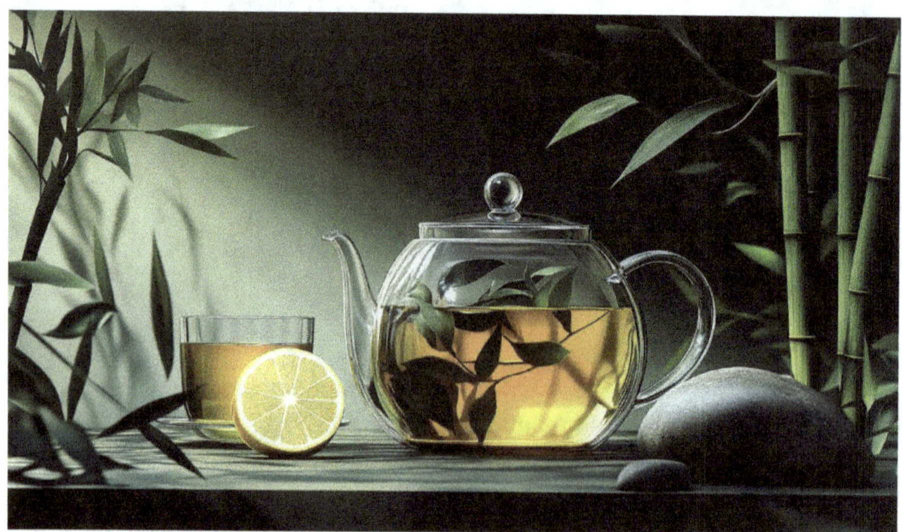

Recipe 64: Gymnema Sylvestre Sugar Cravings Reducer

Gymnema sylvestre, a woody climbing shrub native to India and Africa, has been used in Ayurvedic medicine for centuries. Known as the "sugar destroyer," gymnema leaves contain gymnemic acids, which may help suppress the taste of sweetness and reduce sugar cravings. This herbal infusion offers a natural approach to supporting healthy blood sugar levels and managing appetite.

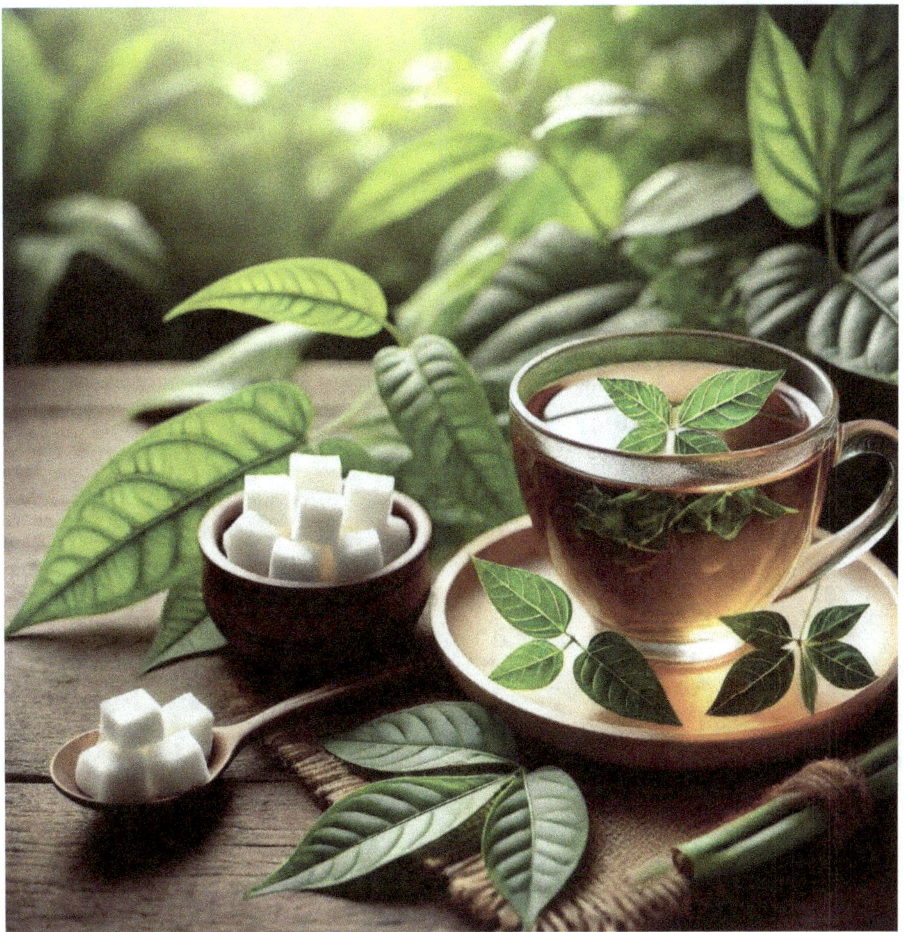

Ingredients:

- 1 teaspoon dried gymnema leaves
- 1 cup boiling water
- Lemon or ginger slice (optional, for flavor)

1. Place the dried gymnema leaves in a teapot or infuser.
2. Pour boiling water over the leaves.
3. Cover and let steep for 5–10 minutes.
4. Strain the infusion into a cup.
5. Add a slice of lemon or ginger if desired to enhance taste.
6. Drink warm.

Usage:

- Consume one cup 30 minutes before meals to help reduce sugar cravings.
- Can be taken once or twice daily.

Caution:

- **Medical Conditions:** If you have diabetes or are on blood sugar-lowering medications, monitor your levels closely and consult a healthcare provider.
- **Pregnancy and Breastfeeding:** Not enough is known about the safety; consult a professional before use.
- **Taste Alteration:** Gymnema may temporarily alter taste perception of sweetness.

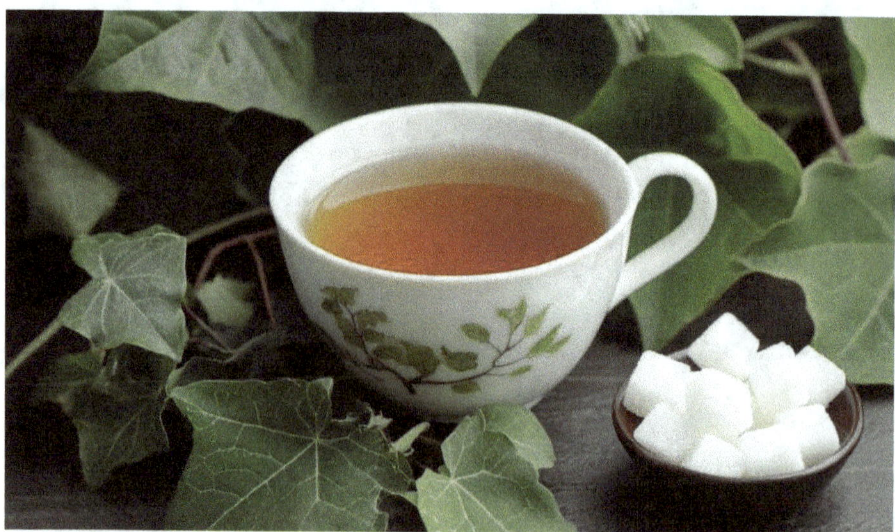

Recipe 65: Hibiscus Blood Pressure Support Tea

Hibiscus flowers, with their vibrant red color, are not only beautiful but also packed with health-promoting properties. Rich in antioxidants like anthocyanins, hibiscus tea has been studied for its potential to support cardiovascular health by helping to lower blood pressure and cholesterol levels. This tart and refreshing tea can be enjoyed hot or cold.

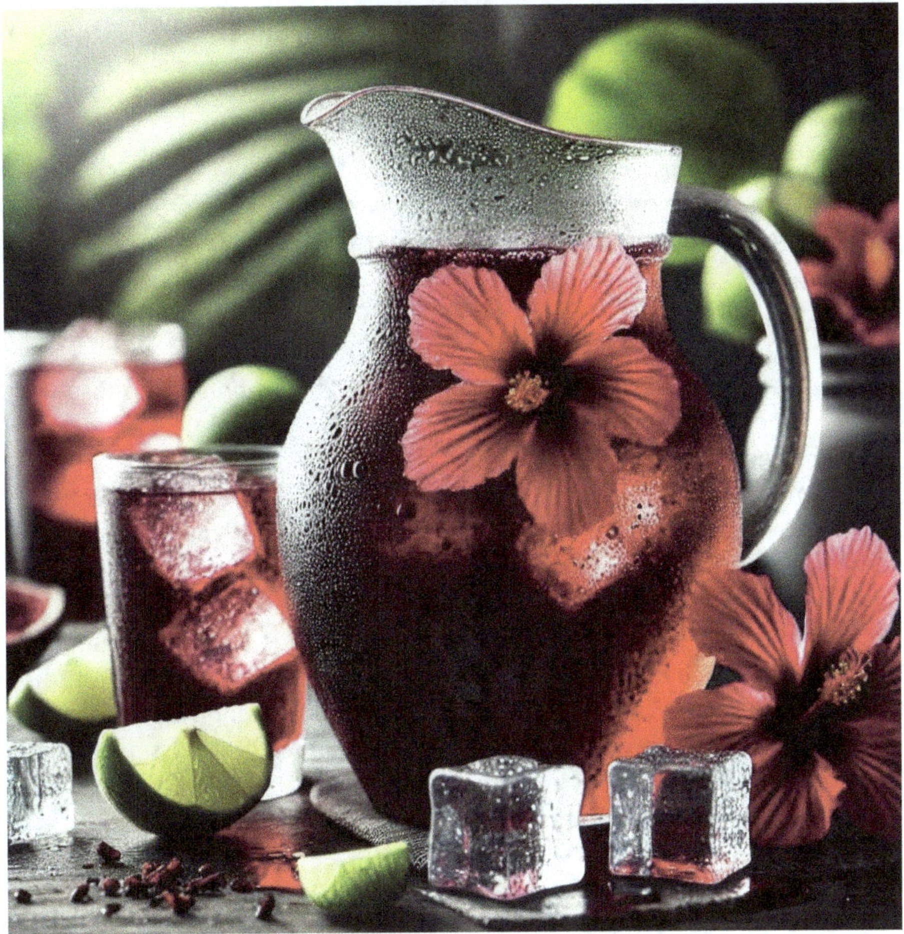

Ingredients:

- 2 tablespoons dried hibiscus petals
- 4 cups water
- Honey or agave syrup (optional, for sweetness)
- Lime or orange slices (optional, for flavor)
- Ice cubes (if serving cold)

Instructions:

1. In a saucepan, bring water to a boil.
2. Remove from heat and add dried hibiscus petals.
3. Cover and steep for 15–20 minutes.
4. Strain the tea into a pitcher, removing the petals.
5. Stir in sweetener if desired, adjusting to taste.
6. Allow the tea to cool to room temperature.
7. Serve over ice with a slice of lime or orange for added flavor, or enjoy warm.

Usage:

- Drink one to two cups daily to support healthy blood pressure levels.
- Consistency over several weeks may offer the best results.

Caution:

- **Medical Conditions:** Hibiscus may lower blood pressure; those with hypotension should use caution.
- **Pregnancy and Breastfeeding:** Avoid use during pregnancy, as hibiscus may have emmenagogue effects; consult a healthcare provider.
- **Medications:** May interact with certain medications like antihypertensives and antidiabetic drugs.

Note: The herbal remedies in this chapter are intended to support metabolic health as part of a balanced diet and healthy lifestyle. They are not substitutes for professional medical advice, diagnosis, or treatment. Individual responses to herbs can vary. Always consult a qualified healthcare professional before starting any new herbal regimen, especially if you have underlying health conditions, are taking medications, or are pregnant or breastfeeding.

Recipe 66: Chamomile and Honey Soothing Syrup

Chamomile, with its gentle apple-like aroma, has been a trusted herb for soothing restlessness and easing digestive discomfort in children for generations. When combined with the natural sweetness of honey, it becomes a comforting syrup that can help calm nerves and promote restful sleep. This simple remedy is a favorite among parents seeking a natural way to soothe their little ones.

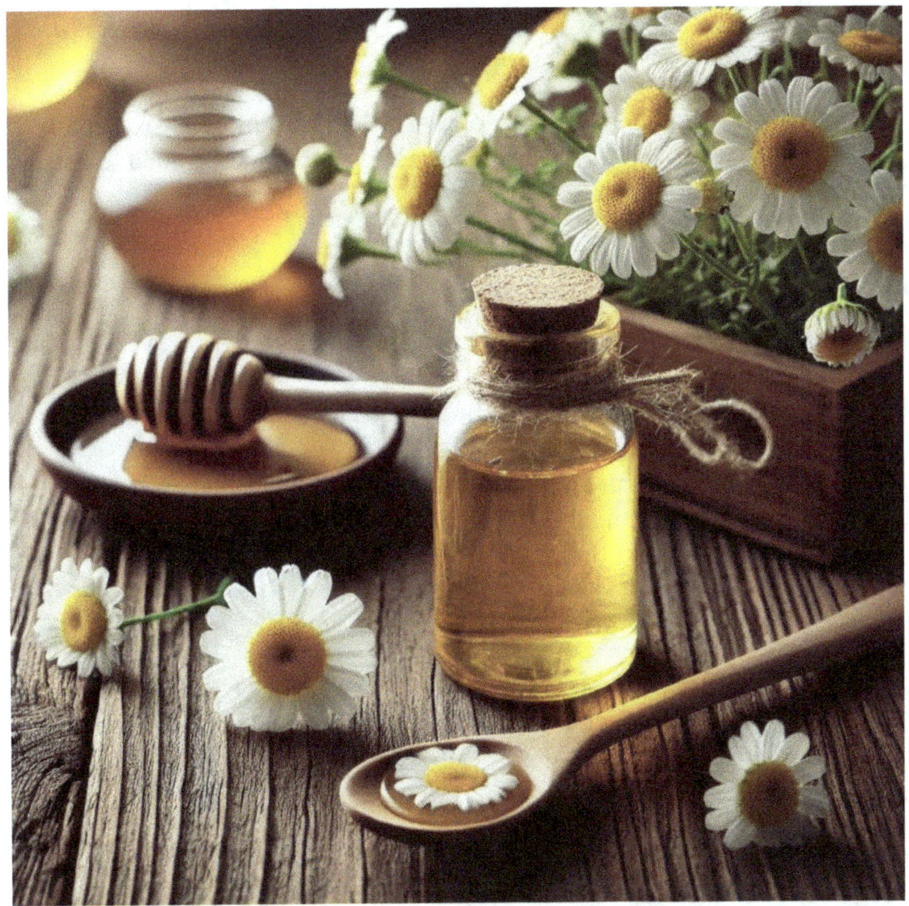

Ingredients:

- 1 cup water
- 2 tablespoons dried chamomile flowers
- ½ cup raw honey (do not give honey to children under one year old)

Instructions:

1. In a small saucepan, bring the water to a boil.
2. Remove from heat and add the dried chamomile flowers.
3. Cover and let steep for 15 minutes.
4. Strain the infusion into a clean bowl, discarding the flowers.
5. While the liquid is still warm (not hot), stir in the raw honey until fully dissolved.
6. Pour the syrup into a sterilized glass bottle with a tight-fitting lid.
7. Label the bottle with the date and contents.
8. Store in the refrigerator for up to two weeks.

Usage:

- For children over one year old, give **1 teaspoon** of the syrup up to three times daily to help soothe restlessness or mild digestive discomfort.

Caution:

- **Honey Warning:** Do not give honey to infants under one year old due to the risk of botulism.
- **Allergies:** Ensure the child is not allergic to chamomile or other plants in the daisy family (Asteraceae).
- **Consult Healthcare Provider:** Always consult a pediatrician before giving herbal remedies to a child, especially if they have underlying health conditions or are taking medications.

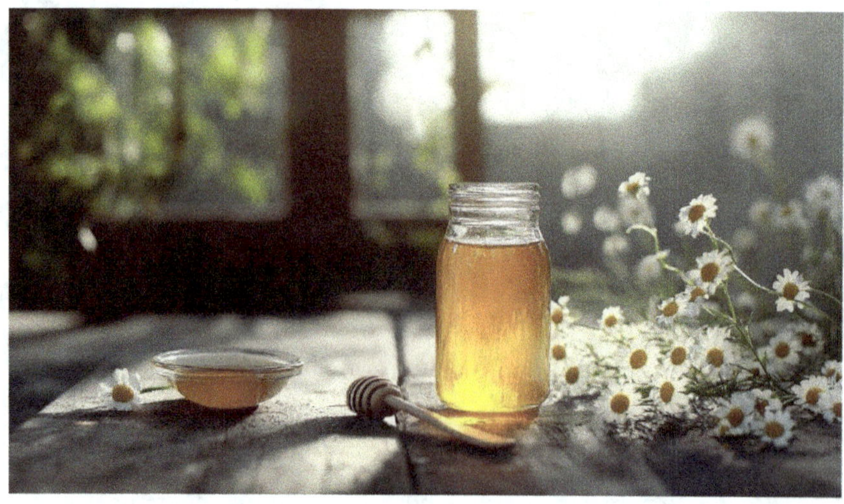

Recipe 67: Marshmallow Root Cough Relief Syrup

Marshmallow root, derived from the marshmallow plant, has been used for centuries to soothe sore throats and ease coughing due to its mucilaginous properties. This gentle herb coats the mucous membranes, providing relief from irritation. Crafting a marshmallow root syrup creates a palatable remedy that can help alleviate coughs in children.

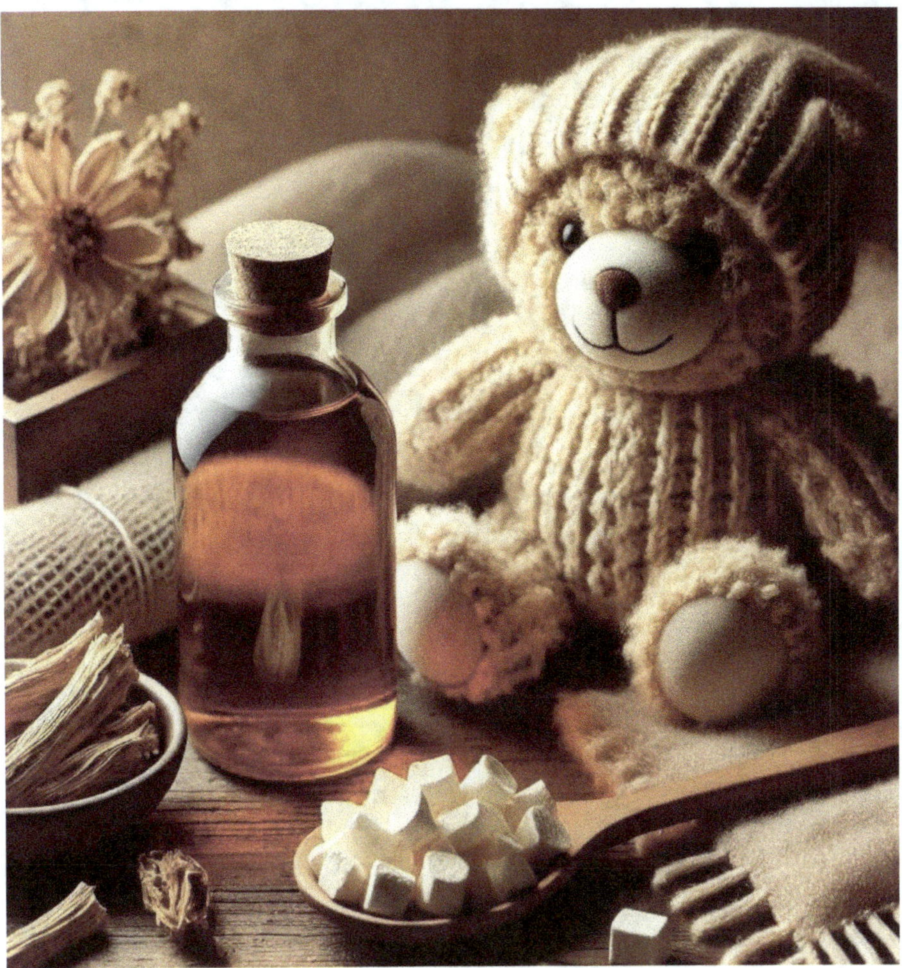

Ingredients:

- 1 cup water
- ¼ cup dried marshmallow root
- ½ cup raw honey (do not give honey to children under one year old)

1. Combine the water and dried marshmallow root in a saucepan.
2. Bring to a gentle simmer over low heat.
3. Cover and let simmer for 15–20 minutes, stirring occasionally.
4. Remove from heat and allow to cool slightly.
5. Strain the mixture through a fine mesh strainer or cheesecloth into a clean bowl.
6. While the liquid is still warm, stir in the raw honey until fully dissolved.
7. Transfer the syrup into a sterilized glass bottle with a lid.
8. Label and date the bottle.
9. Store in the refrigerator for up to two weeks.

Usage:

- For children over one year old, administer **1 teaspoon** of the syrup every 2–3 hours as needed to soothe coughs.

Caution:

- **Honey Warning:** Do not give honey to infants under one year old.
- **Allergies:** Check for potential allergies to marshmallow root.
- **Medical Conditions:** Consult a pediatrician before use, especially if the child has diabetes or is taking medications.

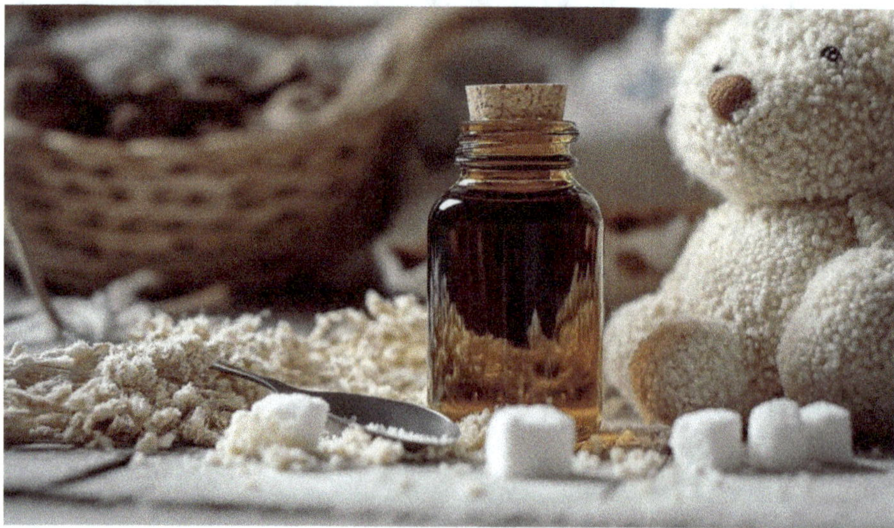

Recipe 68: Lemon Balm Fever-Reducing Popsicles

Lemon balm, with its pleasant lemony scent and taste, is a gentle herb known for its calming effects and mild antiviral properties. When a child has a fever, staying hydrated is crucial. These lemon balm-infused popsicles provide a soothing and enjoyable way to help reduce fever and keep children hydrated.

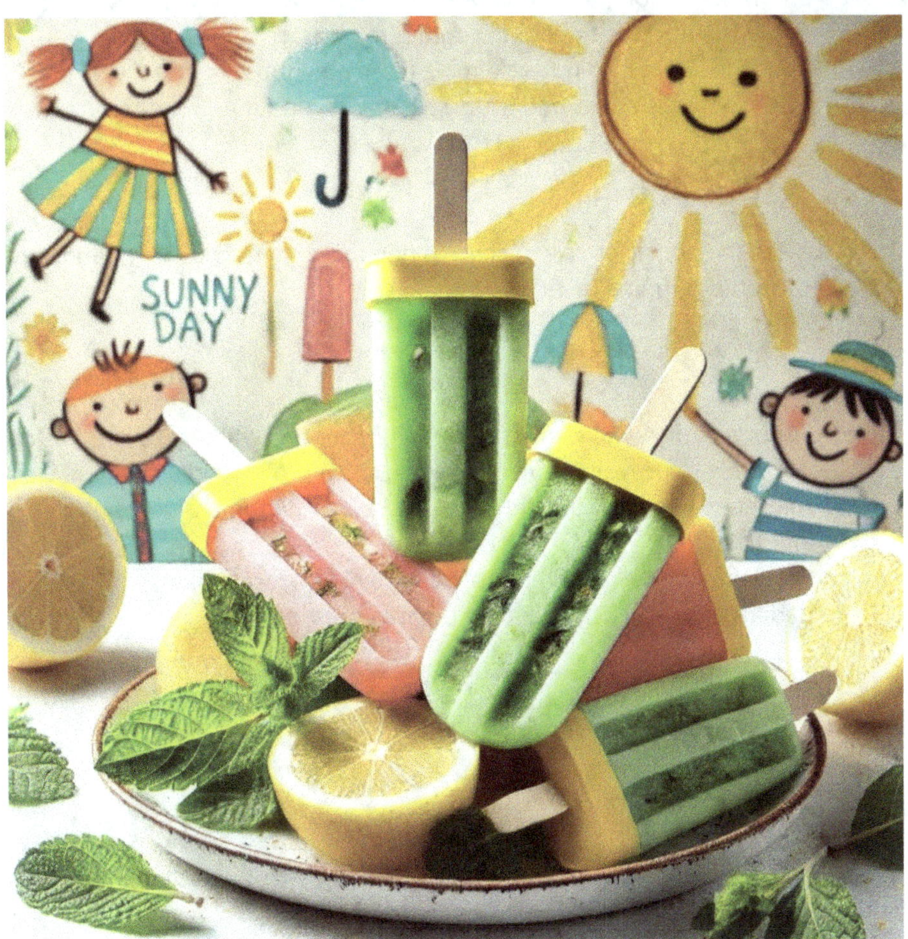

Ingredients:

- 2 cups water
- ¼ cup fresh lemon balm leaves or 2 tablespoons dried leaves
- Juice of one lemon
- 2 tablespoons honey or agave syrup (optional; do not use honey for children under one year old)
- Popsicle molds or small paper cups and popsicle sticks

1. In a saucepan, bring the water to a boil.
2. Remove from heat and add lemon balm leaves.
3. Cover and steep for 15 minutes.
4. Strain the infusion into a bowl, discarding the leaves.
5. Stir in the lemon juice and sweetener if using.
6. Allow the mixture to cool to room temperature.
7. Pour the liquid into popsicle molds or paper cups.
8. Insert popsicle sticks and freeze until solid, about 4–6 hours.

Usage:

- Offer the popsicles to the child as needed to help cool down and stay hydrated during a fever.

Caution:

- **Supervision:** Always supervise young children while they are eating popsicles to prevent choking.
- **Allergies:** Ensure the child is not allergic to lemon balm or any other ingredient.
- **Medical Advice:** A fever can be a sign of serious illness. Consult a pediatrician if the child's fever persists or is high.

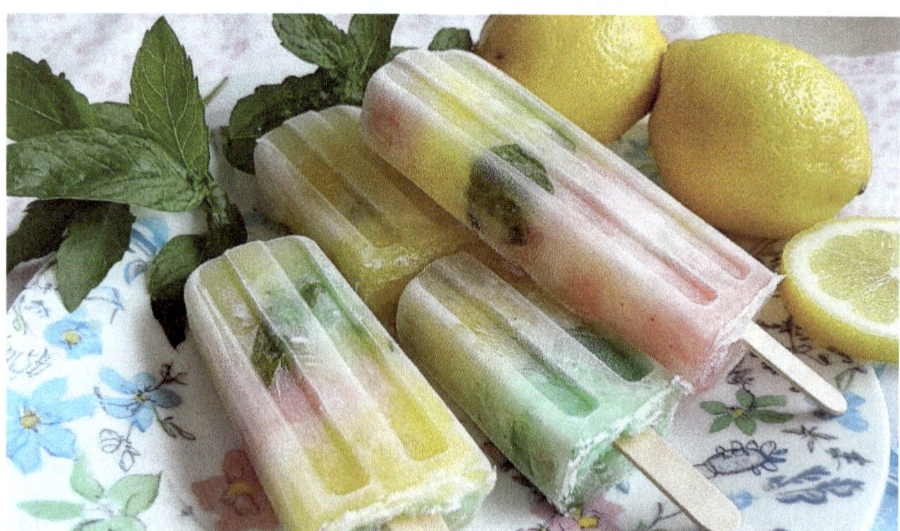

Recipe 69: Catnip Colic Relief Tea

Catnip isn't just for cats; it's a mild herb that can help relieve colic, gas, and restlessness in infants. Its calming properties may soothe the digestive system and promote relaxation. This gentle tea can be given to infants in small amounts or to nursing mothers to pass the benefits through breast milk.

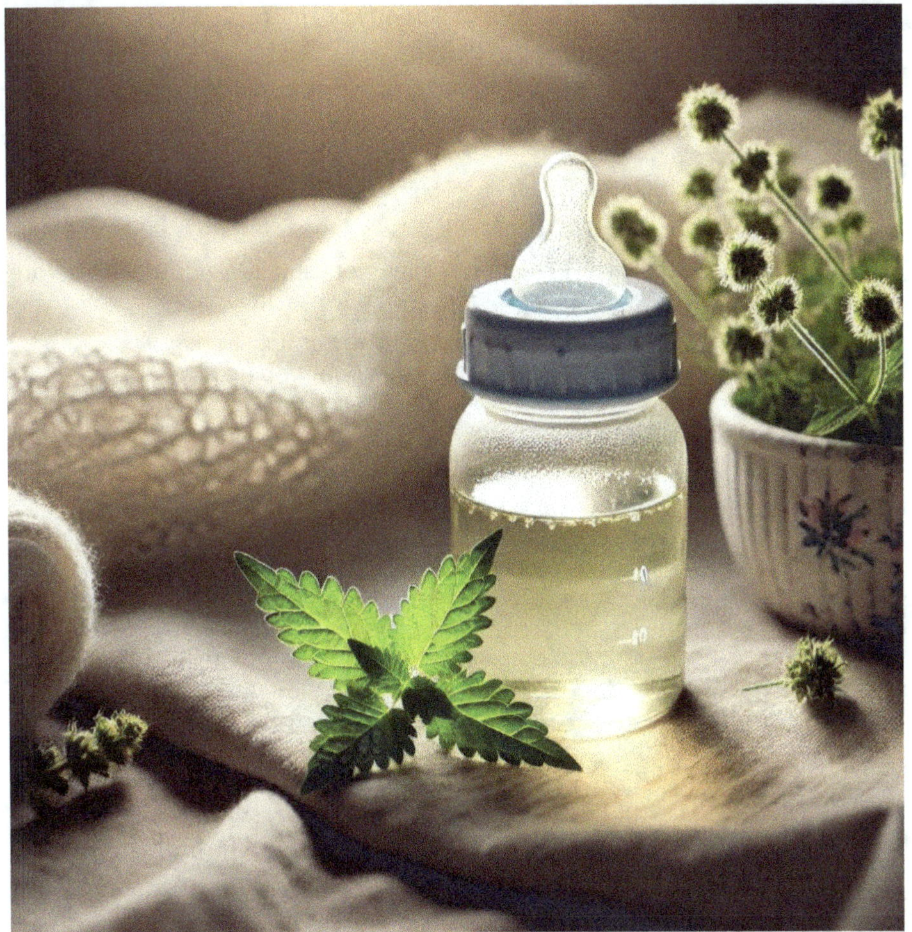

Ingredients:

- 1 teaspoon dried catnip leaves
- 1 cup boiling water

Instructions:

1. Place the dried catnip leaves in a teapot or heatproof mug.

2. Pour boiling water over the herb.
3. Cover and let steep for 10 minutes.
4. Strain the tea into a clean container.
5. Allow the tea to cool completely to room temperature.

- **For Infants:** Administer **1–2 teaspoons** of the cooled tea up to three times daily, using a dropper or baby spoon.
- **For Nursing Mothers:** Drink one cup of the tea 30 minutes before breastfeeding to pass calming effects to the baby.

- **Consult Healthcare Provider:** Always consult a pediatrician before giving herbal remedies to an infant.
- **Allergies:** Check for potential allergies to catnip.
- **Proper Dosage:** Do not exceed the recommended amount for infants.

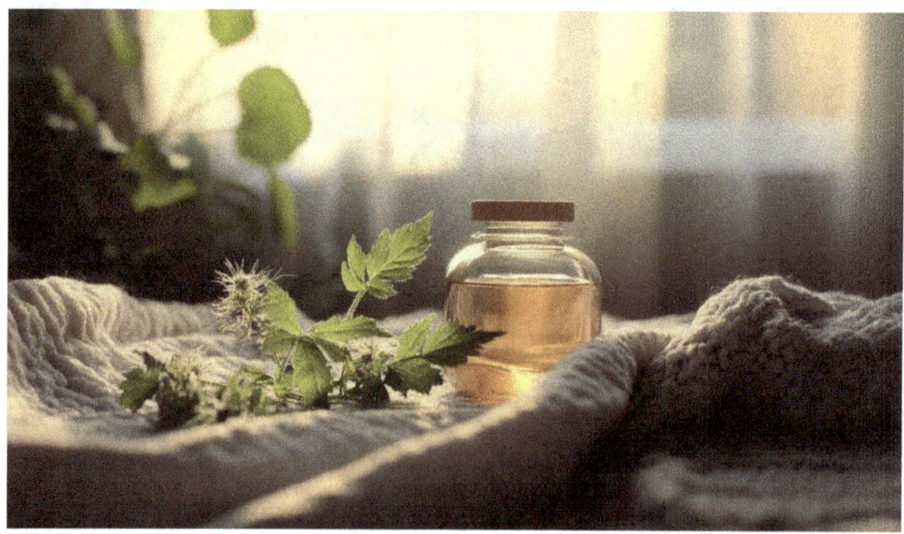

Recipe 70: Elderflower Immune Support Gummies

Elderflowers are known for their immune-boosting properties and pleasant taste, making them suitable for children. Creating gummies with elderflower provides a fun and easy way to support your child's immune system, especially during cold and flu season.

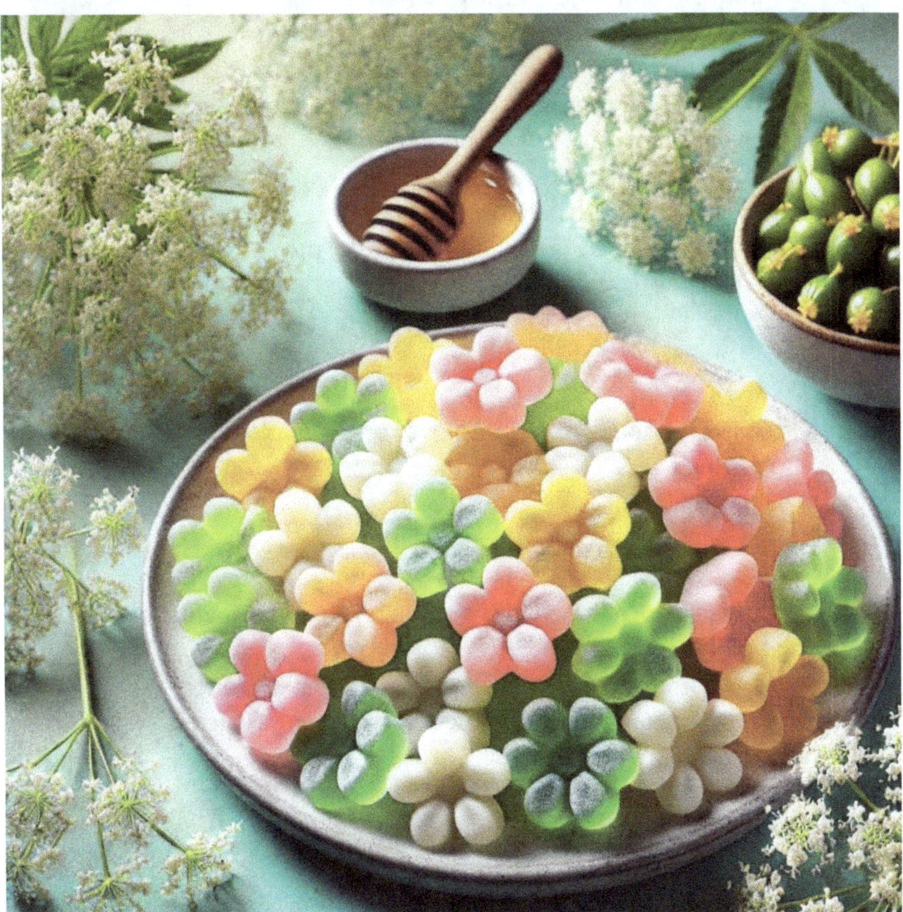

Ingredients:

- 1 cup water
- ¼ cup dried elderflowers
- 2 tablespoons lemon juice
- 2 tablespoons honey or maple syrup (do not use honey for children under one year old)
- 2 tablespoons gelatin powder (use agar-agar for a vegetarian option)
- Silicone gummy molds

1. In a saucepan, bring the water to a boil.
2. Remove from heat and add the dried elderflowers.
3. Cover and let steep for 15 minutes.
4. Strain the infusion into a clean saucepan, discarding the flowers.
5. Stir in the lemon juice and sweetener.
6. Sprinkle the gelatin powder over the warm liquid, stirring constantly until fully dissolved. If using agar-agar, follow package instructions.
7. Gently heat the mixture over low heat if needed to ensure the gelatin dissolves completely, but do not boil.
8. Remove from heat and carefully pour the mixture into silicone molds.
9. Refrigerate for at least 2 hours or until set.
10. Once firm, remove the gummies from the molds.
11. Store in an airtight container in the refrigerator for up to one week.

Usage:

- Offer **1–2 gummies** to children over one year old daily as an immune-supporting treat.

Caution:

- **Allergies:** Ensure the child is not allergic to elderflowers or any other ingredient.
- **Honey Warning:** Do not give honey to infants under one year old.
- **Choking Hazard:** Monitor young children while they consume gummies to prevent choking.
- **Consult Healthcare Provider:** Always consult a pediatrician before giving herbal supplements to a child.

Note: When preparing herbal remedies for children, it is crucial to use age-appropriate dosages and be aware of any potential allergies or contraindications. Always consult a qualified healthcare professional before introducing new herbal remedies to children, especially infants and toddlers. These recipes are intended to support general well-being and are not substitutes for professional medical advice or treatment.

Conclusion

As we reach the end of **"70 Herbal Recipes: Natural Methods of Healing"**, we hope this collection empowers you to embrace the natural remedies that nature provides. Each recipe is crafted to support various aspects of health and wellness, drawing from traditional wisdom and the healing properties of herbs.

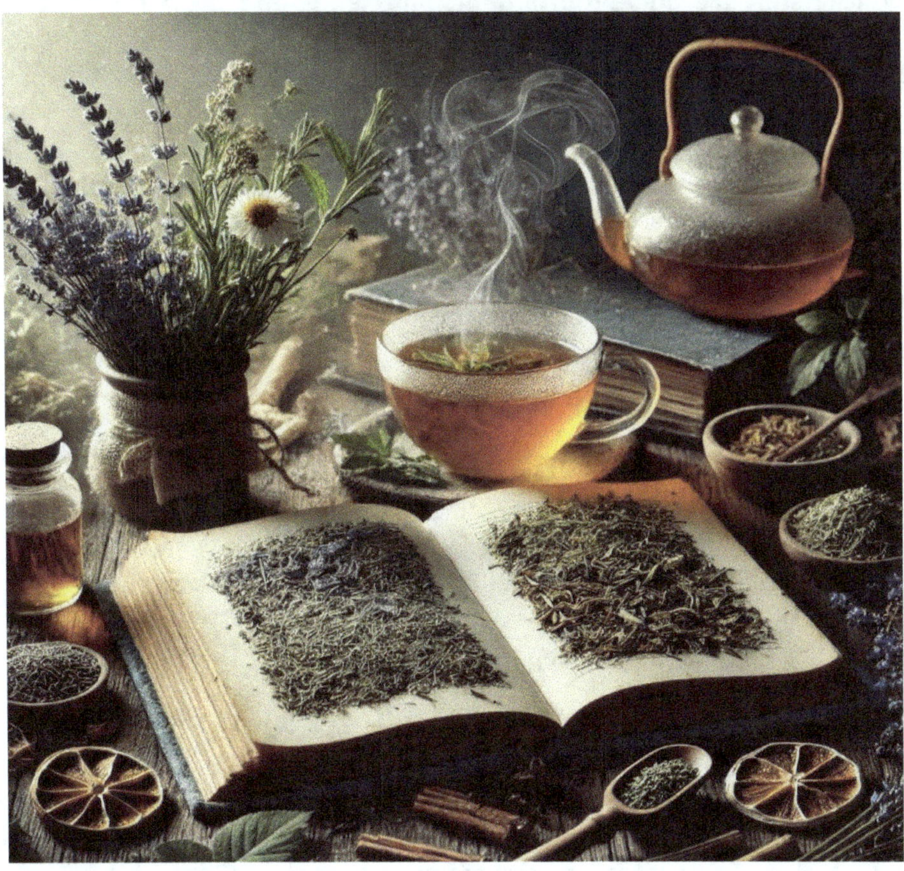

By incorporating these herbal practices into your daily life, you take a step toward holistic well-being, nurturing not just the body but also the mind and spirit. Remember, the journey to health is personal and unique to each individual. Always listen to your body, respect its signals, and consult healthcare professionals when needed.

May this book serve as a trusted companion on your path to natural healing, inspiring you to explore the rich tapestry of herbal traditions and the profound connections between nature and wellness.

Herbs by Health Benefits

In this section, you'll find a quick reference guide that aligns common ailments with the herbs and recipes detailed in this book. Use this guide to identify which herbs may support your specific health needs. Always remember to consult with a healthcare professional before starting any new herbal regimen.

Quick Reference Guide for Ailments and Remedies

Boosting Immunity

- **Echinacea**: Enhances immune response (Recipe 1)
- **Elderberry**: Rich in antioxidants; supports cold prevention (Recipe 2)
- **Garlic**: Natural antibiotic properties; fights infections (Recipe 3)
- **Turmeric**: Anti-inflammatory; supports immune function (Recipe 4)
- **Astragalus**: Adaptogen; strengthens defenses (Recipe 5)

Enhancing Digestion

- **Ginger**: Relieves nausea; aids digestion (Recipe 6)
- **Peppermint**: Eases indigestion and gas (Recipe 7)
- **Fennel**: Reduces bloating; promotes digestion (Recipe 8)
- **Chamomile**: Soothes the stomach; calms the digestive tract (Recipe 9)
- **Dandelion**: Supports liver health; acts as a diuretic (Recipe 10)

Promoting Relaxation and Sleep

- **Lavender**: Calms nerves; promotes restful sleep (Recipe 11)
- **Valerian Root**: Natural sedative; aids in sleep (Recipe 12)
- **Passionflower**: Reduces anxiety; improves sleep quality (Recipe 13)
- **Lemon Balm**: Alleviates stress; uplifts mood (Recipe 14)
- **Hops**: Soothes restlessness; promotes deep sleep (Recipe 15)

Respiratory Health

- **Mullein**: Soothes the respiratory tract; aids in cough relief (Recipe 16)
- **Thyme**: Antimicrobial; clears congestion (Recipe 17)
- **Eucalyptus**: Opens airways; eases breathing (Recipe 18)
- **Licorice Root**: Soothes sore throats; reduces inflammation (Recipe 19)
- **Sage**: Antiseptic; alleviates throat discomfort (Recipe 20)

Skin and Hair Care

- **Aloe Vera**: Heals skin; moisturizes (Recipe 21)
- **Calendula**: Antiseptic; promotes skin repair (Recipe 22)
- **Rosemary**: Strengthens hair; stimulates growth (Recipe 23)
- **Nettle**: Nourishes hair; supports growth (Recipe 24)
- **Tea Tree Oil**: Antibacterial; treats acne (Recipe 25)

Women's Health

- **Red Raspberry Leaf**: Tones the uterus; eases menstrual cramps (Recipe 26)
- **Chasteberry**: Balances hormones; supports menstrual health (Recipe 27)
- **Dong Quai**: Alleviates menstrual discomfort; supports hormonal balance (Recipe 28)
- **Evening Primrose Oil**: Reduces PMS symptoms; supports skin health (Recipe 29)
- **Motherwort**: Calms anxiety; supports menopausal transitions (Recipe 30)

Men's Health

- **Saw Palmetto**: Supports prostate health; reduces urinary symptoms (Recipe 31)
- **Ginseng**: Enhances energy; improves stamina (Recipe 32)
- **Nettle Root**: Promotes urinary health; supports prostate function (Recipe 33)
- **Horny Goat Weed**: Enhances vitality; supports libido (Recipe 34)
- **Pumpkin Seed Oil**: Nourishes prostate; provides essential fatty acids (Recipe 35)

Circulatory Support

- **Hawthorn Berry**: Strengthens the heart; improves circulation (Recipe 36)
- **Ginkgo Biloba**: Enhances blood flow; supports cognitive function (Recipe 37)
- **Cayenne Pepper**: Stimulates circulation; reduces blood clots (Recipe 38)
- **Ginger and Garlic**: Improves cardiovascular health; lowers cholesterol (Recipe 39)

- **Bilberry**: Supports eye health; strengthens capillaries (Recipe 40)

Pain Relief

- **White Willow Bark**: Natural analgesic; reduces inflammation (Recipe 41)
- **Arnica**: Alleviates muscle aches; heals bruises (Recipe 42)
- **Devil's Claw**: Eases joint pain; reduces inflammation (Recipe 43)
- **St. John's Wort**: Soothes nerve pain; promotes healing (Recipe 44)
- **Turmeric**: Anti-inflammatory; relieves joint pain (Recipe 45)

Energy and Vitality

- **Maca Root**: Boosts energy; balances hormones (Recipe 46)
- **Ashwagandha**: Reduces stress; enhances vitality (Recipe 47)
- **Rhodiola**: Fights fatigue; improves endurance (Recipe 48)
- **Holy Basil (Tulsi)**: Balances energy; reduces stress (Recipe 49)
- **Schisandra Berry**: Enhances stamina; supports liver health (Recipe 50)

Detoxification

- **Milk Thistle**: Protects liver; aids detoxification (Recipe 51)
- **Burdock Root**: Purifies blood; supports skin health (Recipe 52)
- **Dandelion and Nettle**: Diuretic; cleanses the body (Recipe 53)
- **Cilantro and Parsley**: Binds heavy metals; supports elimination (Recipe 54)
- **Lemon and Ginger**: Stimulates digestion; supports detox (Recipe 55)

Cognitive Support

- **Rosemary**: Improves memory; enhances alertness (Recipe 56)
- **Bacopa Monnieri**: Supports brain function; enhances learning (Recipe 57)
- **Gotu Kola**: Promotes mental clarity; reduces anxiety (Recipe 58)
- **Sage**: Boosts cognition; supports memory (Recipe 59)
- **Lemon Balm**: Enhances focus; uplifts mood (Recipe 60)

Metabolic Health

- **Cinnamon and Clove**: Regulates blood sugar; supports metabolism (Recipe 61)

- **Fenugreek Seed**: Improves insulin function; reduces cholesterol (Recipe 62)
- **Green Tea**: Antioxidant-rich; boosts metabolism (Recipe 63)
- **Gymnema Sylvestre**: Reduces sugar cravings; supports glucose levels (Recipe 64)
- **Hibiscus**: Lowers blood pressure; supports heart health (Recipe 65)

Children's Remedies

- **Chamomile**: Calms restlessness; soothes digestion (Recipe 66)
- **Marshmallow Root**: Eases coughs; soothes sore throats (Recipe 67)
- **Lemon Balm**: Reduces fever; calms nerves (Recipe 68)
- **Catnip**: Relieves colic; promotes relaxation (Recipe 69)
- **Elderflower**: Supports immunity; gentle antiviral (Recipe 70)

Cultivating your own herbs is a rewarding way to ensure you have a fresh, organic supply for your remedies. Whether you have a spacious garden or a small windowsill, you can grow a variety of herbs suited to your space and climate.

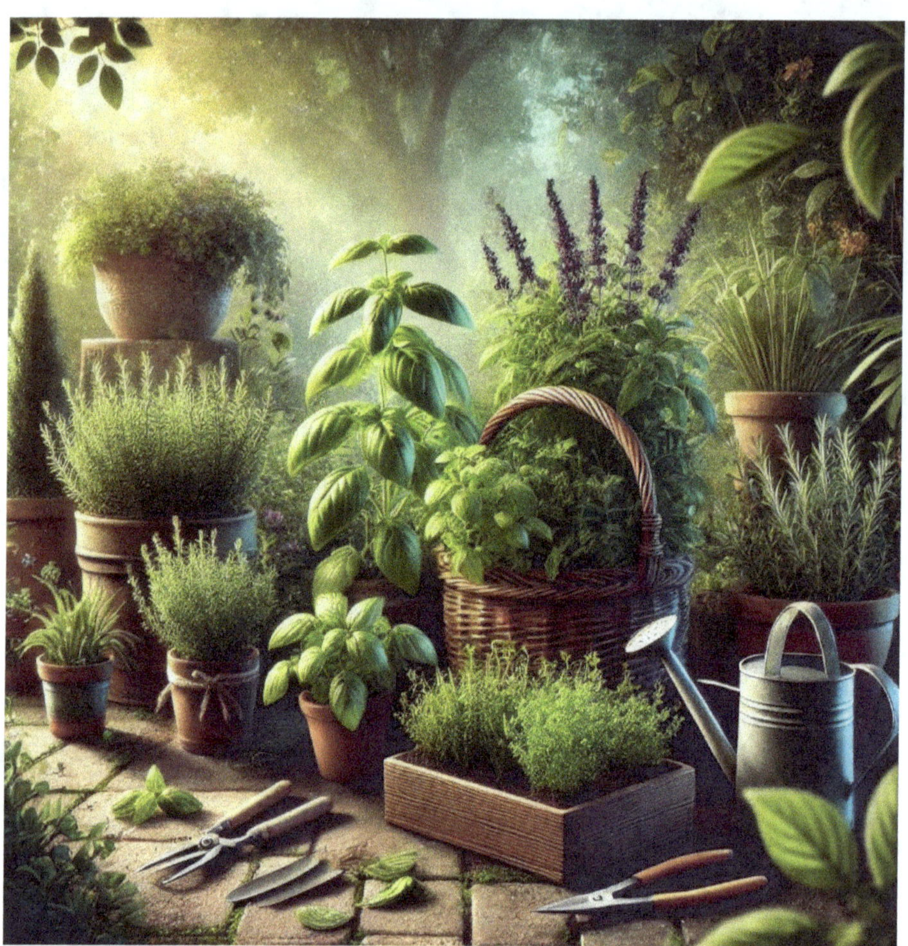

Starting Your Herb Garden

1. Planning Your Garden

- **Assess Your Space**: Determine how much space you have—garden beds, pots, or window boxes.
- **Sunlight Requirements**: Most herbs need at least 6 hours of sunlight daily.

- **Climate Considerations**: Choose herbs that thrive in your local climate.

2. Selecting Herbs to Grow

- **Beginner-Friendly Herbs**: Basil, mint, parsley, and chives are easy to grow.
- **Medicinal Herbs**: Consider planting chamomile, lavender, echinacea, and calendula.
- **Perennials vs. Annuals**: Perennials like sage and thyme return yearly; annuals like basil need replanting.

Soil Preparation and Planting

1. Soil Quality

- **Well-Draining Soil**: Herbs prefer soil that doesn't retain excess water.
- **Soil Enrichment**: Add organic compost to provide nutrients.
- **pH Level**: Most herbs thrive in slightly acidic to neutral soil (pH 6.0–7.0).

2. Planting Techniques

- **Seeds vs. Seedlings**: Seeds are economical; seedlings offer a head start.
- **Spacing**: Allow enough space for growth; overcrowding can hinder development.
- **Watering**: Water thoroughly after planting; maintain consistent moisture without overwatering.

Sustainable Harvesting Practices

1. Ethical Harvesting

- **Respect Plant Life**: Harvest without damaging the plant's ability to regrow.
- **Seasonal Timing**: Harvest herbs at their peak potency, usually just before flowering.
- **Rotating Harvests**: Avoid depleting any one area or plant.

2. Harvesting Techniques

- **Use Sharp Tools**: Clean cuts prevent plant damage and disease.
- **Morning Harvest**: Essential oils are most concentrated in the morning after dew evaporates.
- **Leafy Herbs**: Harvest leaves from the top to encourage bushier growth.

1. Drying Methods

- **Air Drying**: Bundle herbs and hang upside down in a warm, dry place.
- **Dehydrator**: Use a food dehydrator set to low heat.
- **Oven Drying**: Spread herbs on a baking sheet; dry at the lowest temperature with the door slightly open.

2. Storing Dried Herbs

- **Containers**: Use airtight glass jars to preserve freshness.
- **Labeling**: Include the herb name and harvest date.
- **Storage Conditions**: Keep in a cool, dark place away from sunlight and moisture.

Making Herbal Preparations

Understanding different herbal preparation methods allows you to maximize the benefits of the herbs you grow or purchase. This section guides you through creating various forms of herbal remedies.

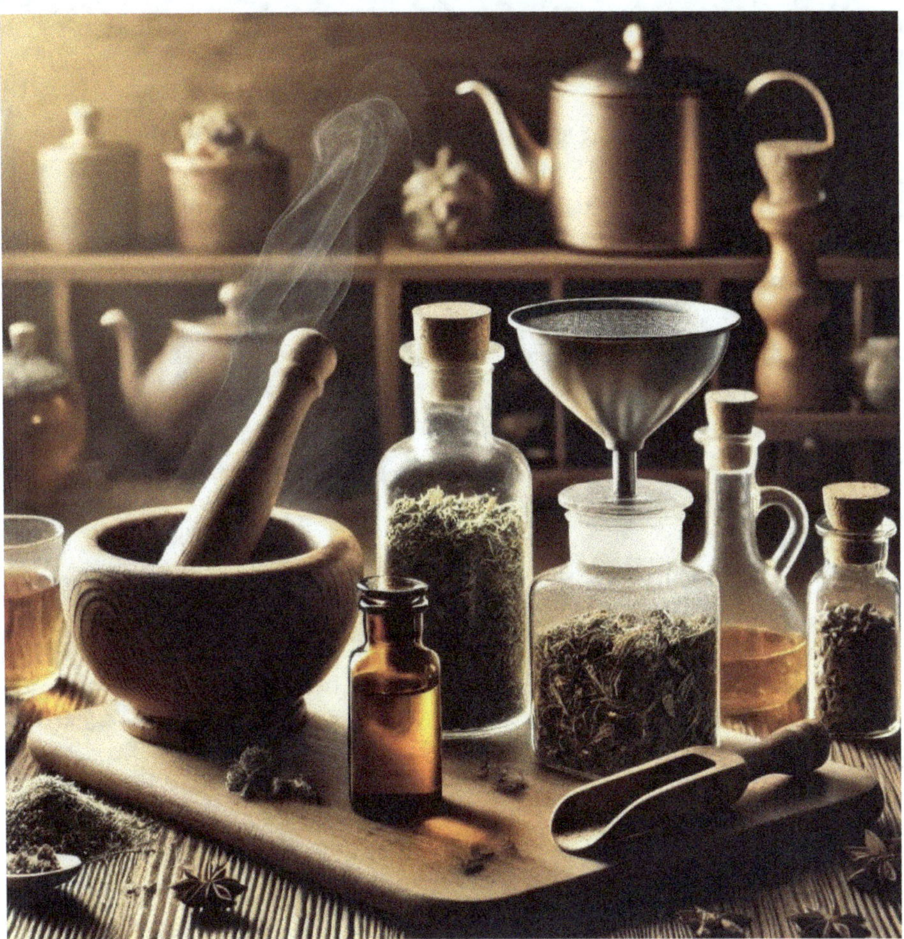

Understanding Herbal Forms

- **Teas and Infusions**: Ideal for extracting water-soluble compounds from leaves and flowers.
- **Decoctions**: Used for tougher plant materials like roots and bark.
- **Tinctures**: Alcohol or glycerin-based extracts that preserve herbs and concentrate their properties.
- **Salves and Ointments**: Topical preparations combining herbs with oils and beeswax.

- **Syrups and Elixirs**: Sweetened herbal extracts, often used for coughs and sore throats.
- **Capsules and Powders**: Ground herbs encapsulated for convenient ingestion.

Techniques for Teas and Infusions

1. Basic Herbal Tea

- **Ratio**: Typically, 1 teaspoon of dried herb per cup of water.
- **Steeping Time**: 5–15 minutes, depending on the herb.
- **Covering**: Always cover while steeping to retain volatile oils.

2. Infusions

- **Overnight Infusions**: For stronger medicinal effects, steep herbs overnight.
- **Herb Quantity**: Use more herb, about 1 ounce per quart of water.

Crafting Tinctures and Extracts

1. Alcohol-Based Tinctures

- **Solvent Choice**: Use vodka or brandy (40–50% alcohol).
- **Herb-to-Solvent Ratio**: Generally, 1 part herb to 5 parts alcohol.
- **Extraction Time**: Steep for 4–6 weeks in a dark place, shaking occasionally.

2. Glycerin-Based Extracts

- **For Alcohol-Free Preparations**: Use vegetable glycerin.
- **Dilution**: Mix glycerin with distilled water (60% glycerin to 40% water).
- **Process**: Similar to alcohol tinctures, but may require gentle heating.

Creating Salves and Ointments

1. Herbal Oils

- **Infusion**: Steep herbs in a carrier oil (olive, almond) using sunlight or gentle heat.

- **Timeframe**: Solar infusion takes 4–6 weeks; heat infusion takes a few hours.

2. Making Salves

- **Ingredients**: Combine infused oil with beeswax.
- **Ratio**: Approximately 1 cup oil to ¼ cup beeswax.
- **Process**: Melt beeswax, mix with oil, pour into containers, and let cool.

Preparing Syrups and Elixirs

1. Herbal Syrups

- **Base**: Strong herbal decoction.
- **Sweetener**: Add honey or sugar (1 part sweetener to 2 parts liquid).
- **Preservation**: Store in the refrigerator; can last several weeks.

2. Elixirs

- **Combination**: Blend tinctures with honey or glycerin for a palatable remedy.
- **Customization**: Add spices or citrus zest for flavor and added benefits.

Making Capsules and Powders

- **Drying Herbs**: Ensure herbs are thoroughly dried before grinding.
- **Grinding**: Use a mortar and pestle or coffee grinder to create a fine powder.
- **Encapsulation**: Fill capsules using a capsule machine or by hand.
- **Storage**: Keep capsules in airtight containers away from light and moisture.

Glossary of Herbs

An alphabetical list of the herbs mentioned in this book, including their botanical names, descriptions, primary uses, and precautions.

A

- **Ashwagandha (Withania somnifera)**
  - *Description*: A root used as an adaptogen in Ayurvedic medicine.
  - *Uses*: Reduces stress, enhances vitality.
  - *Precautions*: Consult a healthcare provider if you have thyroid issues.

B

- **Bacopa Monnieri (Bacopa monnieri)**
  - *Description*: A creeping herb used in Ayurveda.
  - *Uses*: Supports cognitive function and memory.
  - *Precautions*: May cause digestive discomfort.

C

- **Calendula (Calendula officinalis)**
  - *Description*: A bright orange or yellow flowering plant often used for skin conditions.
  - *Uses*: Promotes wound healing, soothes irritated skin, and reduces inflammation.
  - *Precautions*: Generally safe for topical use; avoid if allergic to plants in the Asteraceae family.
- **Catnip (Nepeta cataria)**
  - *Description*: A mint-family herb known for its calming effects on humans and stimulating effects on cats.
  - *Uses*: Relieves colic, promotes relaxation, and supports digestion.
  - *Precautions*: Avoid excessive use in children and during pregnancy.
- **Chamomile (Matricaria chamomilla or Chamaemelum nobile)**
  - *Description*: A small, daisy-like flower with a mild, apple-like scent.

- o *Uses*: Calms anxiety, promotes sleep, and soothes the digestive tract.
  - o *Precautions*: Avoid if allergic to ragweed or related plants.
- **Chasteberry (Vitex agnus-castus)**
  - o *Description*: A fruit-bearing shrub used in traditional medicine for hormonal health.
  - o *Uses*: Balances hormones, supports menstrual health, and reduces PMS symptoms.
  - o *Precautions*: May interfere with hormone therapies or birth control.

D

- **Dandelion (Taraxacum officinale)**
  - o *Description*: A common weed with yellow flowers and deeply toothed leaves, rich in vitamins and minerals.
  - o *Uses*: Supports liver health, acts as a diuretic, and aids digestion.
  - o *Precautions*: May interact with diuretics or medications for high blood pressure.
- **Devil's Claw (Harpagophytum procumbens)**
  - o *Description*: A root native to southern Africa, named for its hooked fruit.
  - o *Uses*: Alleviates joint pain, reduces inflammation, and supports mobility.
  - o *Precautions*: Not recommended for individuals with stomach ulcers or gallstones.
- **Dong Quai (Angelica sinensis)**
  - o *Description*: A root used in Traditional Chinese Medicine, often called "female ginseng."
  - o *Uses*: Balances hormones, supports menstrual health, and alleviates menopausal symptoms.
  - o *Precautions*: Avoid during pregnancy or if taking blood thinners.

E

- **Echinacea (Echinacea purpurea or E. angustifolia)**
  - o *Description*: A purple coneflower native to North America, valued for its immune-boosting properties.
  - o *Uses*: Enhances immune response, reduces cold symptoms, and fights infections.

- o *Precautions*: Avoid if allergic to ragweed or related plants; prolonged use may decrease effectiveness.
- **Elderberry (Sambucus nigra)**
  - o *Description*: A dark purple berry from the elder tree, rich in antioxidants.
  - o *Uses*: Supports the immune system, alleviates cold and flu symptoms, and reduces inflammation.
  - o *Precautions*: Raw berries and other parts of the plant can be toxic if not cooked properly.
- **Evening Primrose (Oenothera biennis)**
  - o *Description*: A plant with yellow flowers, its seeds are used for their oil, rich in gamma-linolenic acid (GLA).
  - o *Uses*: Reduces PMS symptoms, supports skin health, and alleviates joint pain.
  - o *Precautions*: May interact with anticoagulants or anti-seizure medications.

G

- **Garlic (Allium sativum)**
  - o *Description*: A pungent bulb widely used in cooking and medicine.
  - o *Uses*: Natural antibiotic, supports heart health, and boosts immunity.
  - o *Precautions*: May thin blood; consult a doctor before use with anticoagulants or before surgery.
- **Ginger (Zingiber officinale)**
  - o *Description*: A spicy root commonly used to relieve nausea and improve digestion.
  - o *Uses*: Eases motion sickness, reduces inflammation, and supports digestion.
  - o *Precautions*: High doses may cause heartburn; consult a healthcare provider if pregnant.
- **Ginkgo Biloba (Ginkgo biloba)**
  - o *Description*: One of the oldest tree species, valued for its brain-boosting properties.
  - o *Uses*: Enhances memory, improves circulation, and supports cognitive health.
  - o *Precautions*: May interact with blood thinners and should be avoided before surgery.
- **Gotu Kola (Centella asiatica)**

- o *Description*: A creeping herb used in Ayurvedic and Traditional Chinese Medicine.
  - o *Uses*: Improves concentration, reduces anxiety, and promotes wound healing.
  - o *Precautions*: May affect liver enzymes; consult a doctor if you have liver conditions.

H

- **Hawthorn (Crataegus monogyna or C. oxyacantha)**
  - o *Description*: A small tree with white flowers and red berries, used for heart health.
  - o *Uses*: Strengthens the heart, improves circulation, and reduces blood pressure.
  - o *Precautions*: May interact with heart medications; consult a healthcare provider before use.
- **Hibiscus (Hibiscus sabdariffa)**
  - o *Description*: A tropical flower with vibrant red petals, often used in teas.
  - o *Uses*: Lowers blood pressure, supports liver health, and provides antioxidants.
  - o *Precautions*: May lower blood pressure; avoid use during pregnancy.
- **Holy Basil (Ocimum sanctum or O. tenuiflorum)**
  - o *Description*: A fragrant herb revered in Ayurvedic medicine, also called Tulsi.
  - o *Uses*: Reduces stress, balances energy, and supports respiratory health.
  - o *Precautions*: May lower blood sugar; monitor levels if diabetic.

L

- **Lavender (Lavandula angustifolia)**
  - o *Description*: A fragrant flowering plant widely used for relaxation.
  - o *Uses*: Calms anxiety, improves sleep, and soothes headaches.
  - o *Precautions*: Rarely, lavender oil may cause skin irritation; test before topical use.
- **Lemon Balm (Melissa officinalis)**
  - o *Description*: A lemon-scented herb in the mint family, known for its calming effects.
  - o *Uses*: Reduces anxiety, supports sleep, and enhances mood.

- o *Precautions*: May interfere with thyroid function; consult a doctor if you have thyroid issues.
- **Licorice Root (Glycyrrhiza glabra)**
  - o *Description*: A sweet-tasting root used for respiratory and digestive support.
  - o *Uses*: Soothes sore throats, reduces inflammation, and supports adrenal health.
  - o *Precautions*: Prolonged use can raise blood pressure; avoid if hypertensive.

M

- **Maca (Lepidium meyenii)**
  - o *Description*: A root vegetable native to the Andes, often used as a powdered superfood.
  - o *Uses*: Boosts energy, supports hormonal balance, and enhances stamina.
  - o *Precautions*: May interfere with hormone-sensitive conditions; consult a doctor before use.
- **Marshmallow Root (Althaea officinalis)**
  - o *Description*: A mucilaginous root used for soothing irritated tissues.
  - o *Uses*: Relieves coughs, soothes sore throats, and supports digestive health.
  - o *Precautions*: May interact with medications by delaying absorption; space doses apart.
- **Milk Thistle (Silybum marianum)**
  - o *Description*: A spiny plant with purple flowers, known for its liver-protecting properties.
  - o *Uses*: Supports liver detoxification, protects liver cells, and reduces inflammation.
  - o *Precautions*: Avoid if allergic to plants in the Asteraceae family.
- **Motherwort (Leonurus cardiaca)**
  - o *Description*: A herbaceous plant in the mint family, often used for women's health.
  - o *Uses*: Reduces anxiety, supports heart health, and eases menopausal symptoms.
  - o *Precautions*: Avoid during pregnancy as it may stimulate uterine contractions.
- **Mullein (Verbascum thapsus)**

- o *Description*: A tall, flowering plant with soft, fuzzy leaves used for respiratory health.
  - o *Uses*: Soothes the lungs, reduces coughs, and clears congestion.
  - o *Precautions*: Avoid if allergic to plants in the figwort family (Scrophulariaceae).

N

- **Nettle (Urtica dioica)**
  - o *Description*: A nutrient-rich herb often used for skin, hair, and overall vitality.
  - o *Uses*: Supports hair growth, reduces inflammation, and promotes urinary health.
  - o *Precautions*: Handle fresh leaves with care; they may sting. Cooking or drying neutralizes the sting.

P

- **Passionflower (Passiflora incarnata)**
  - o *Description*: A climbing vine with intricate flowers, used for its calming properties.
  - o *Uses*: Reduces anxiety, promotes restful sleep, and eases nervous tension.
  - o *Precautions*: May cause drowsiness; avoid combining with sedatives.
- **Peppermint (Mentha × piperita)**
  - o *Description*: A hybrid mint with a refreshing aroma and cooling properties.
  - o *Uses*: Eases indigestion, relieves headaches, and clears nasal congestion.
  - o *Precautions*: Avoid excessive use in children or if you have acid reflux.

R

- **Red Raspberry Leaf (Rubus idaeus)**
  - o *Description*: The leaves of the raspberry plant, commonly used for women's reproductive health.
  - o *Uses*: Tones the uterus, reduces menstrual cramps, and supports pregnancy in later stages.

- o *Precautions*: Consult a healthcare provider before use during early pregnancy.
- **Rhodiola (Rhodiola rosea)**
  - o *Description*: A flowering plant that grows in cold regions, known for its adaptogenic properties.
  - o *Uses*: Reduces fatigue, improves mental clarity, and supports physical endurance.
  - o *Precautions*: May cause dizziness or dry mouth in some individuals.
- **Rosemary (Rosmarinus officinalis)**
  - o *Description*: A woody herb with needle-like leaves and a pungent aroma, often used for cognitive support.
  - o *Uses*: Enhances memory, stimulates circulation, and supports hair growth.
  - o *Precautions*: Avoid in high doses during pregnancy or if you have epilepsy.

S

- **Sage (Salvia officinalis)**
  - o *Description*: A gray-green herb with a strong aroma, often used for digestive and respiratory health.
  - o *Uses*: Boosts cognition, soothes sore throats, and reduces excessive sweating.
  - o *Precautions*: Avoid prolonged use in high doses, as it may cause side effects like dizziness.
- **Saw Palmetto (Serenoa repens)**
  - o *Description*: A small palm tree native to the southeastern United States, used for men's health.
  - o *Uses*: Supports prostate health and reduces urinary symptoms.
  - o *Precautions*: May interact with hormone therapies or blood-thinning medications.
- **Schisandra (Schisandra chinensis)**
  - o *Description*: A berry-producing vine used in Traditional Chinese Medicine for vitality and endurance.
  - o *Uses*: Enhances stamina, supports liver function, and reduces stress.
  - o *Precautions*: May affect liver enzymes; consult a healthcare provider if you have liver conditions.

- **Tea Tree (Melaleuca alternifolia)**
  - *Description*: A small tree native to Australia, valued for its antimicrobial essential oil.
  - *Uses*: Treats acne, soothes minor cuts, and acts as an antifungal.
  - *Precautions*: For external use only; may cause irritation in sensitive individuals.
- **Thyme (Thymus vulgaris)**
  - *Description*: A low-growing herb with small, fragrant leaves, often used for respiratory health.
  - *Uses*: Clears congestion, soothes coughs, and acts as a natural antiseptic.
  - *Precautions*: Avoid in high doses during pregnancy, as it may stimulate uterine contractions.
- **Turmeric (Curcuma longa)**
  - *Description*: A bright yellow root used for its anti-inflammatory and antioxidant properties.
  - *Uses*: Reduces joint pain, supports liver health, and boosts immunity.
  - *Precautions*: High doses may cause stomach upset; consult a doctor if you have gallbladder issues.

V

- **Valerian (Valeriana officinalis)**
  - *Description*: A flowering plant with a pungent root often used for sleep and relaxation.
  - *Uses*: Promotes restful sleep, reduces anxiety, and eases nervous tension.
  - *Precautions*: May cause drowsiness; avoid combining with alcohol or sedatives.

W

- **White Willow (Salix alba)**
  - *Description*: A tree with bark that contains salicin, a natural precursor to aspirin.
  - *Uses*: Reduces pain, alleviates headaches, and soothes inflammation.
  - *Precautions*: Avoid if allergic to aspirin or salicylates.

- **Yarrow (Achillea millefolium)**
  - o *Description*: A flowering plant traditionally used for wound care and digestive health.
  - o *Uses*: Stops bleeding, reduces inflammation, and soothes indigestion.
  - o *Precautions*: Avoid during pregnancy, as it may stimulate uterine contractions.

Thank You

Thank you for embarking on this herbal journey. May the knowledge and recipes within empower you to embrace natural methods of healing and enrich your life with the gifts of nature.